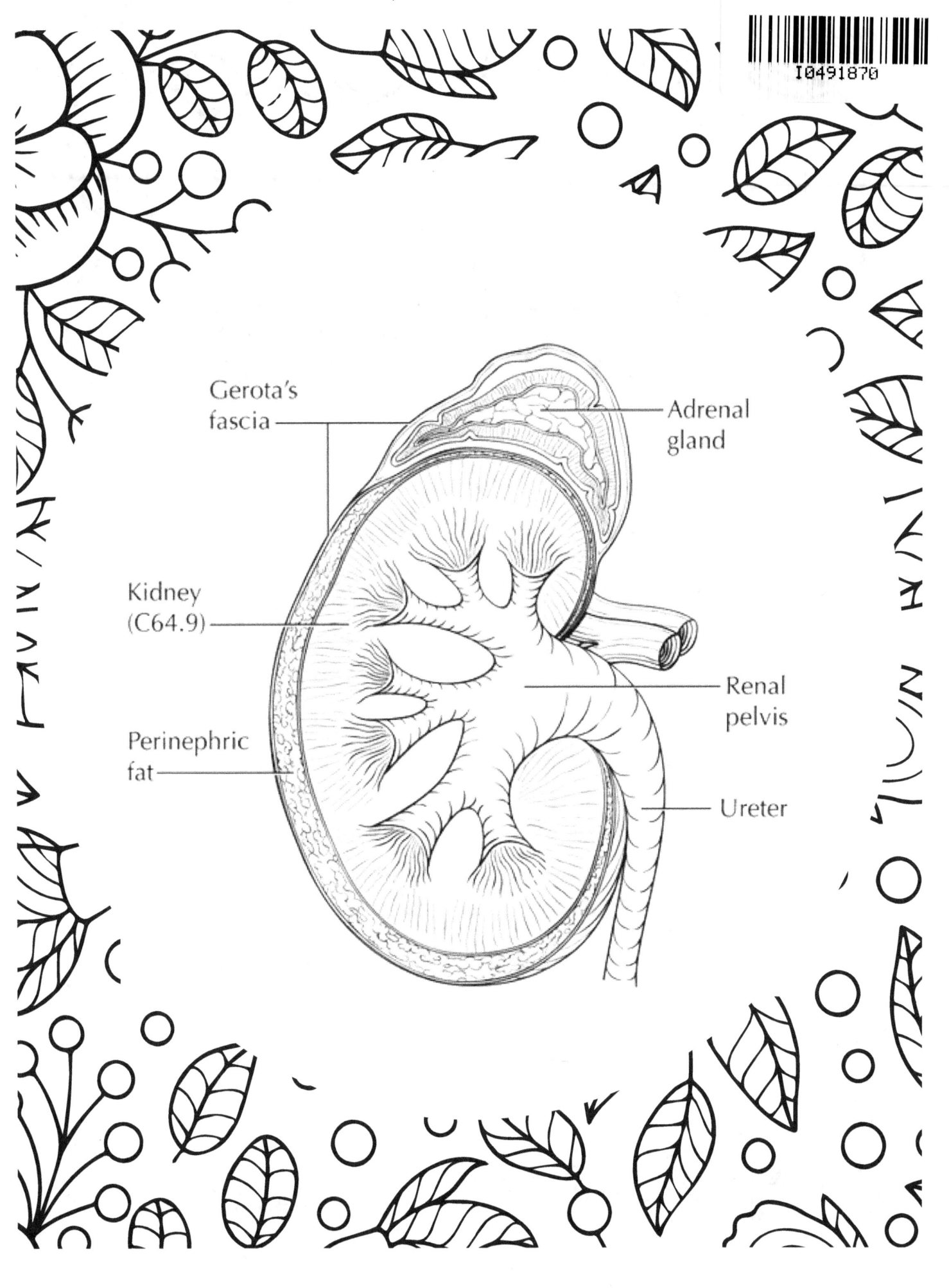

Gerota's fascia

Adrenal gland

Kidney (C64.9)

Renal pelvis

Perinephric fat

Ureter

This Book Belongs To

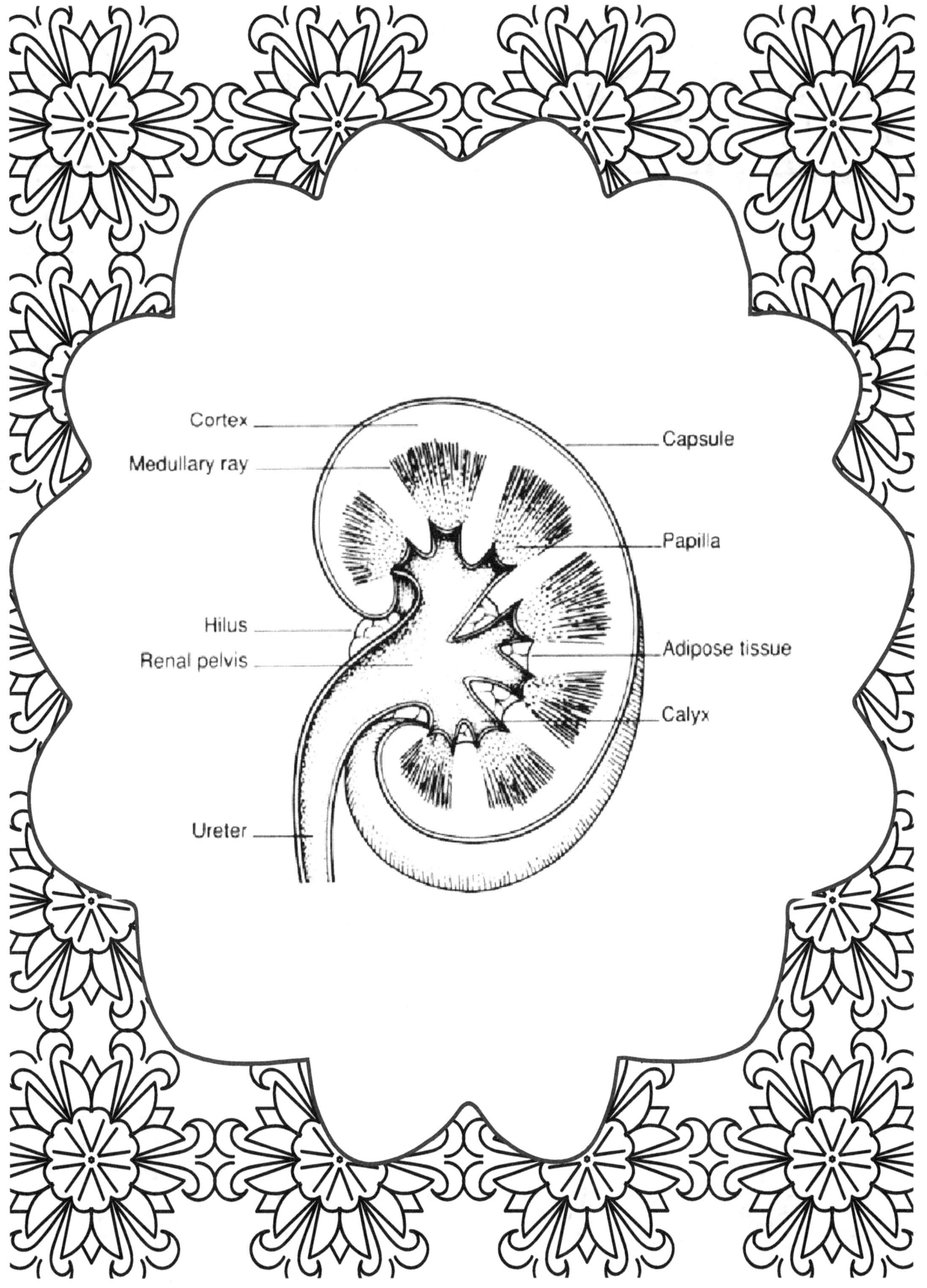

Cortex

Medullary ray

Hilus

Renal pelvis

Ureter

Capsule

Papilla

Adipose tissue

Calyx

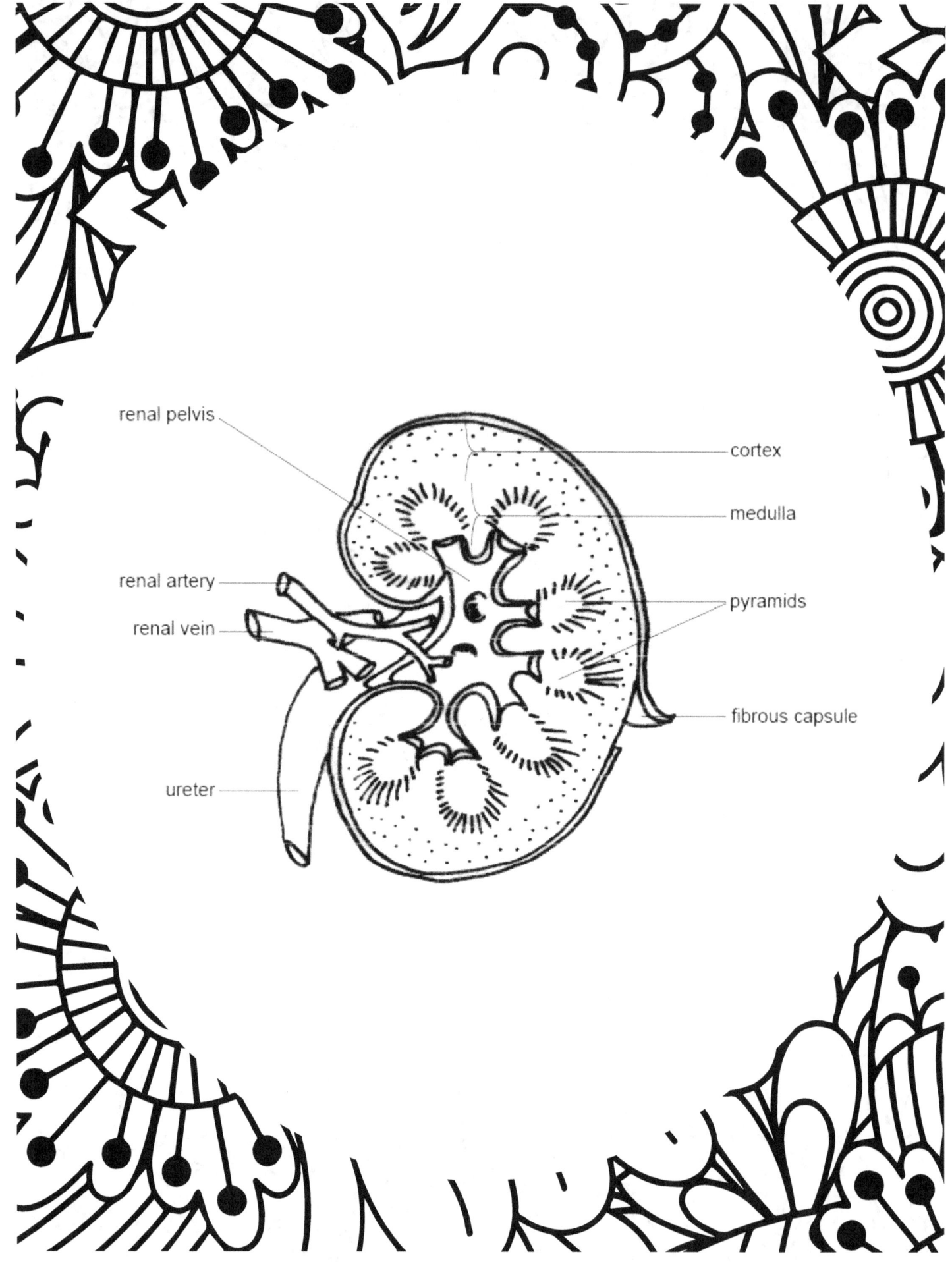

renal pelvis

cortex

medulla

renal artery

renal vein

pyramids

ureter

fibrous capsule

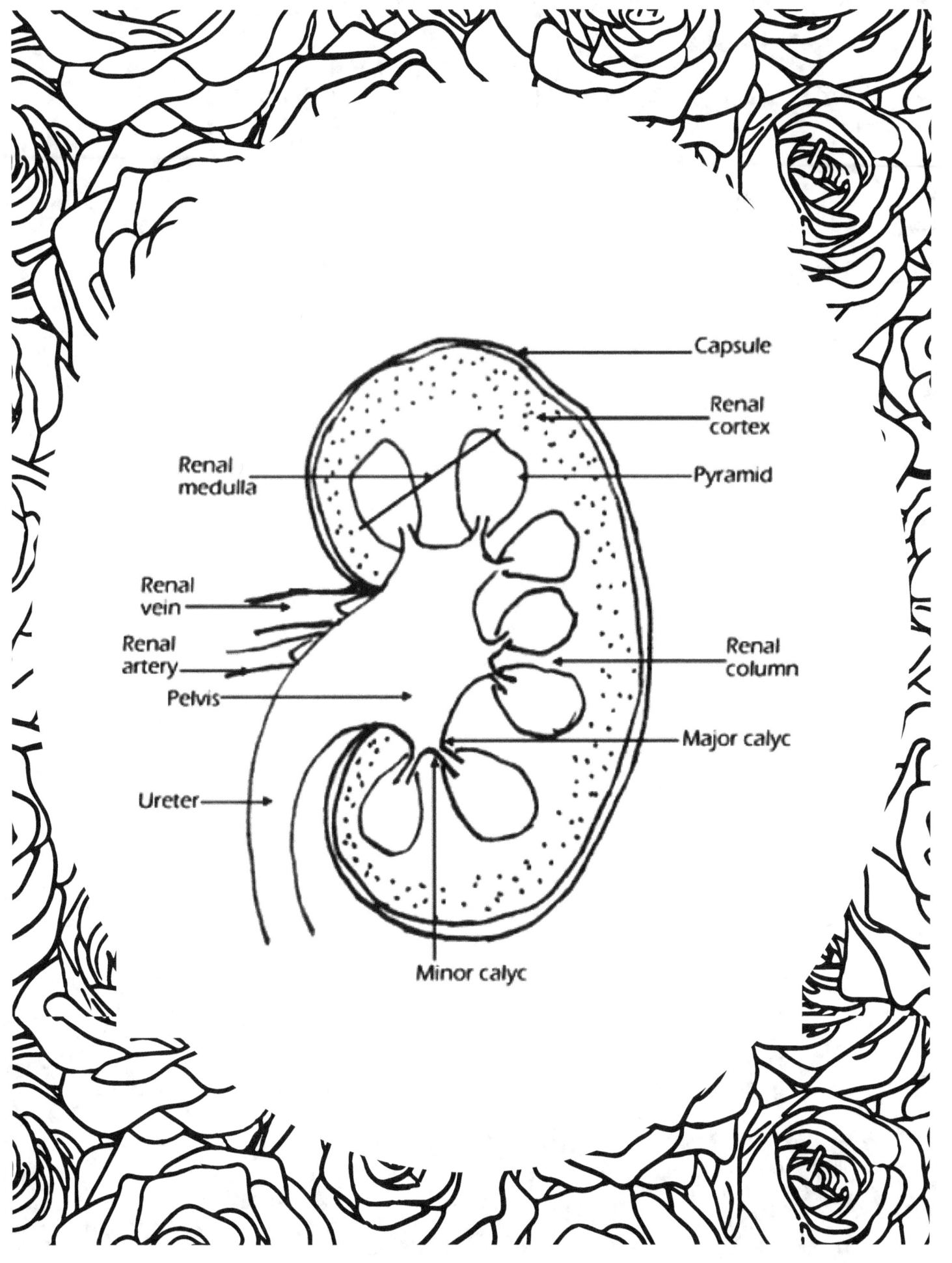

Capsule

Renal cortex

Pyramid

Renal medulla

Renal vein

Renal artery

Pelvis

Renal column

Major calyc

Ureter

Minor calyc

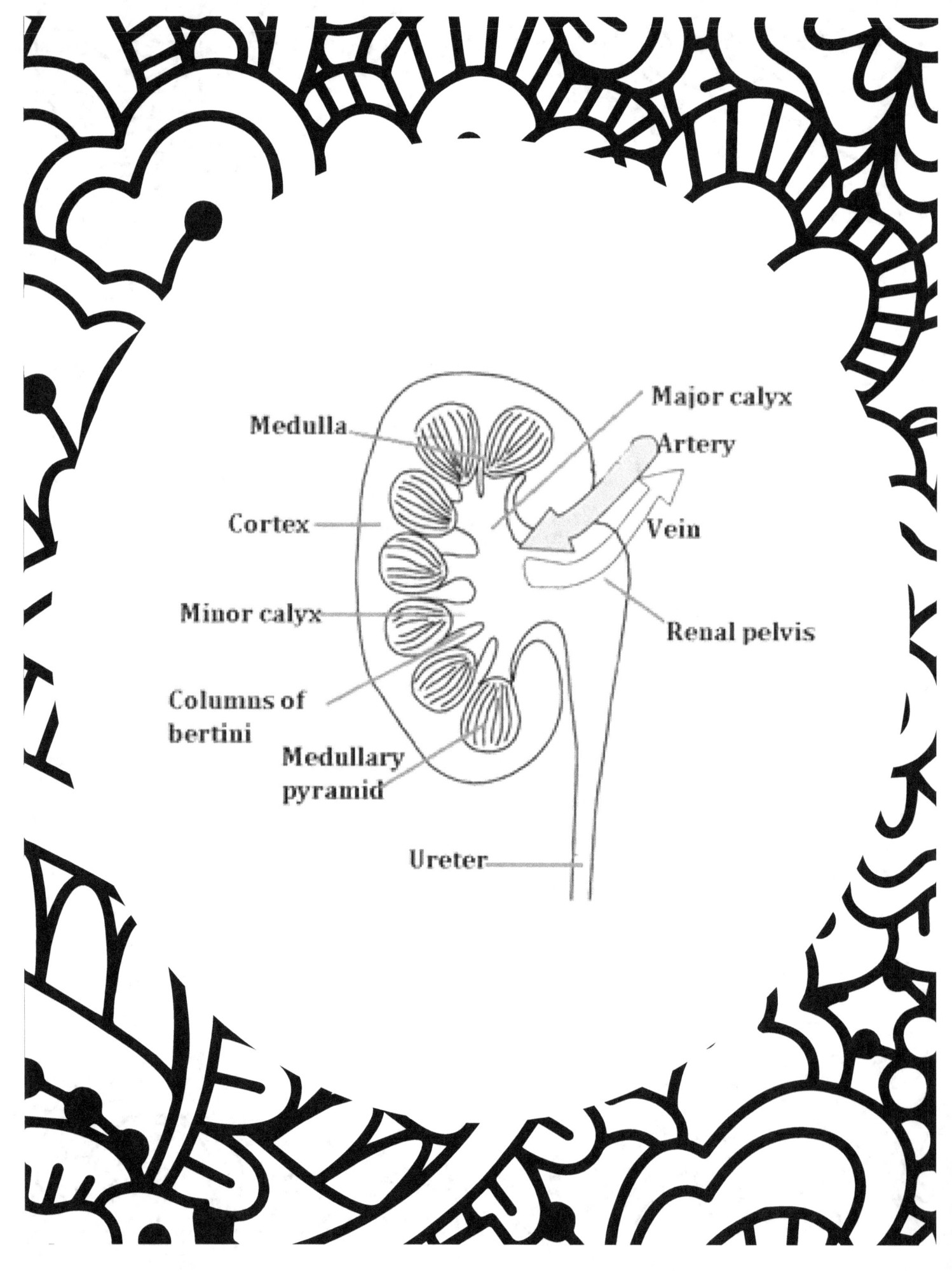

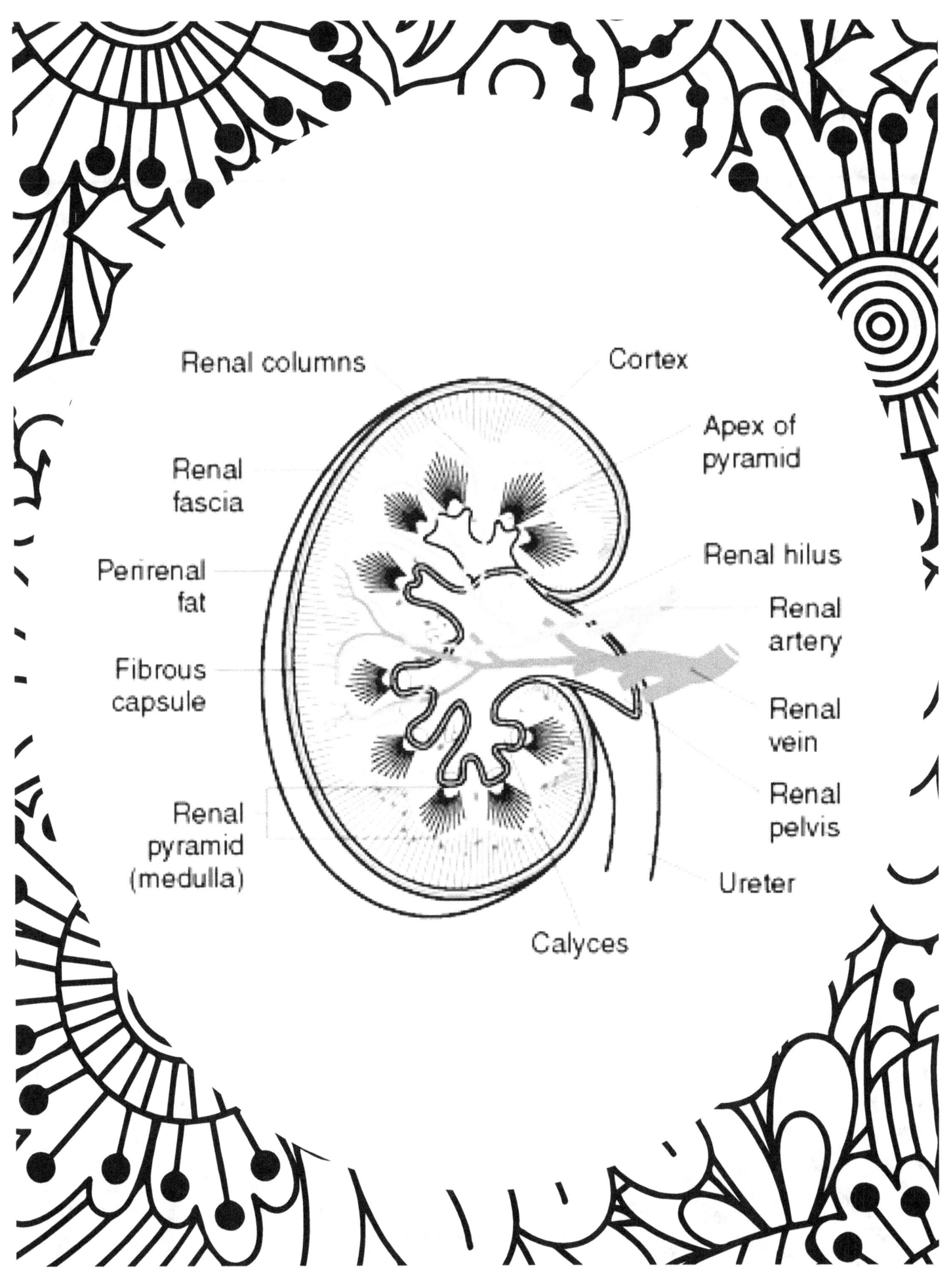

Renal columns

Cortex

Renal fascia

Apex of pyramid

Perirenal fat

Renal hilus

Renal artery

Fibrous capsule

Renal vein

Renal pelvis

Renal pyramid (medulla)

Ureter

Calyces

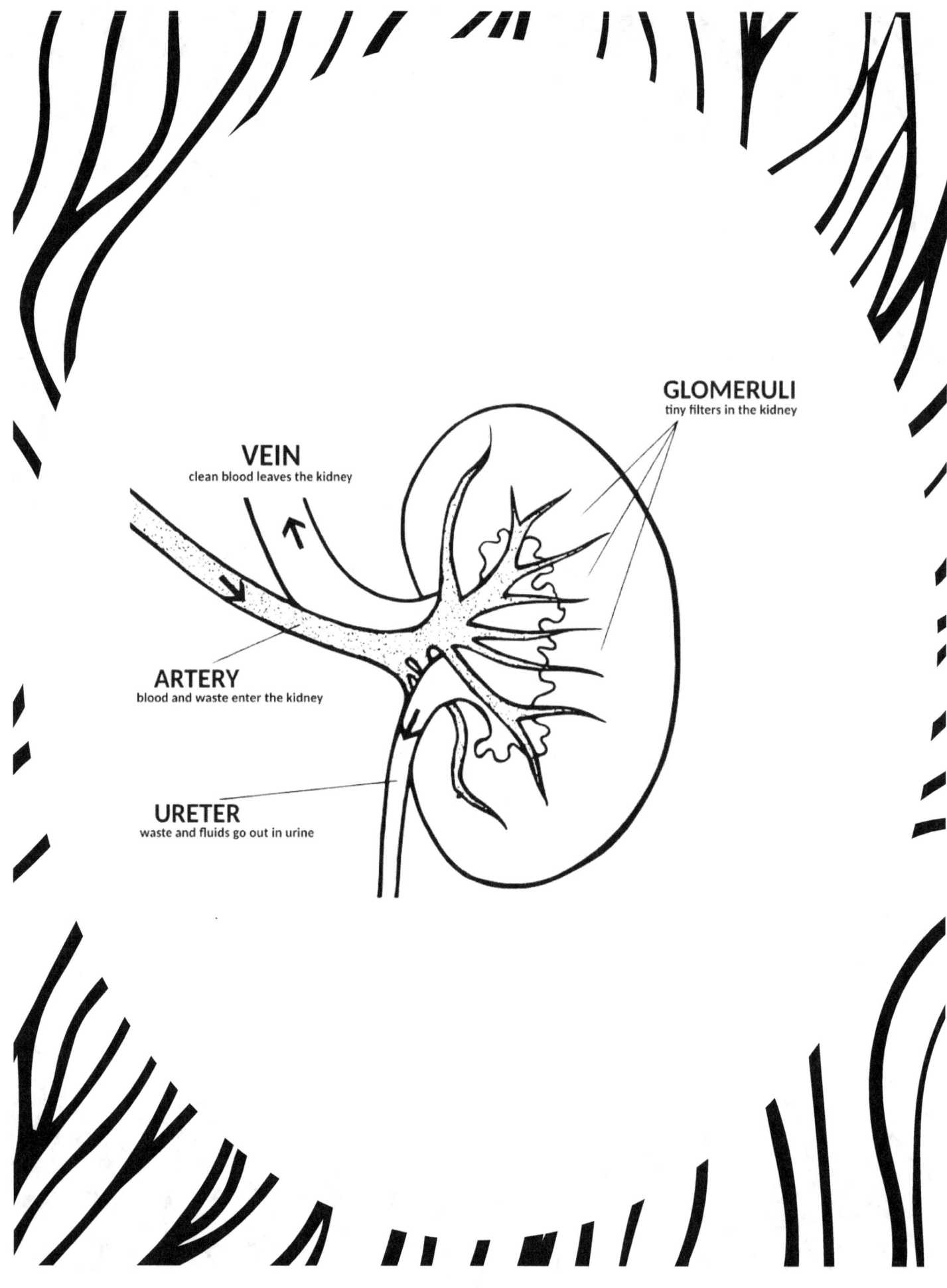

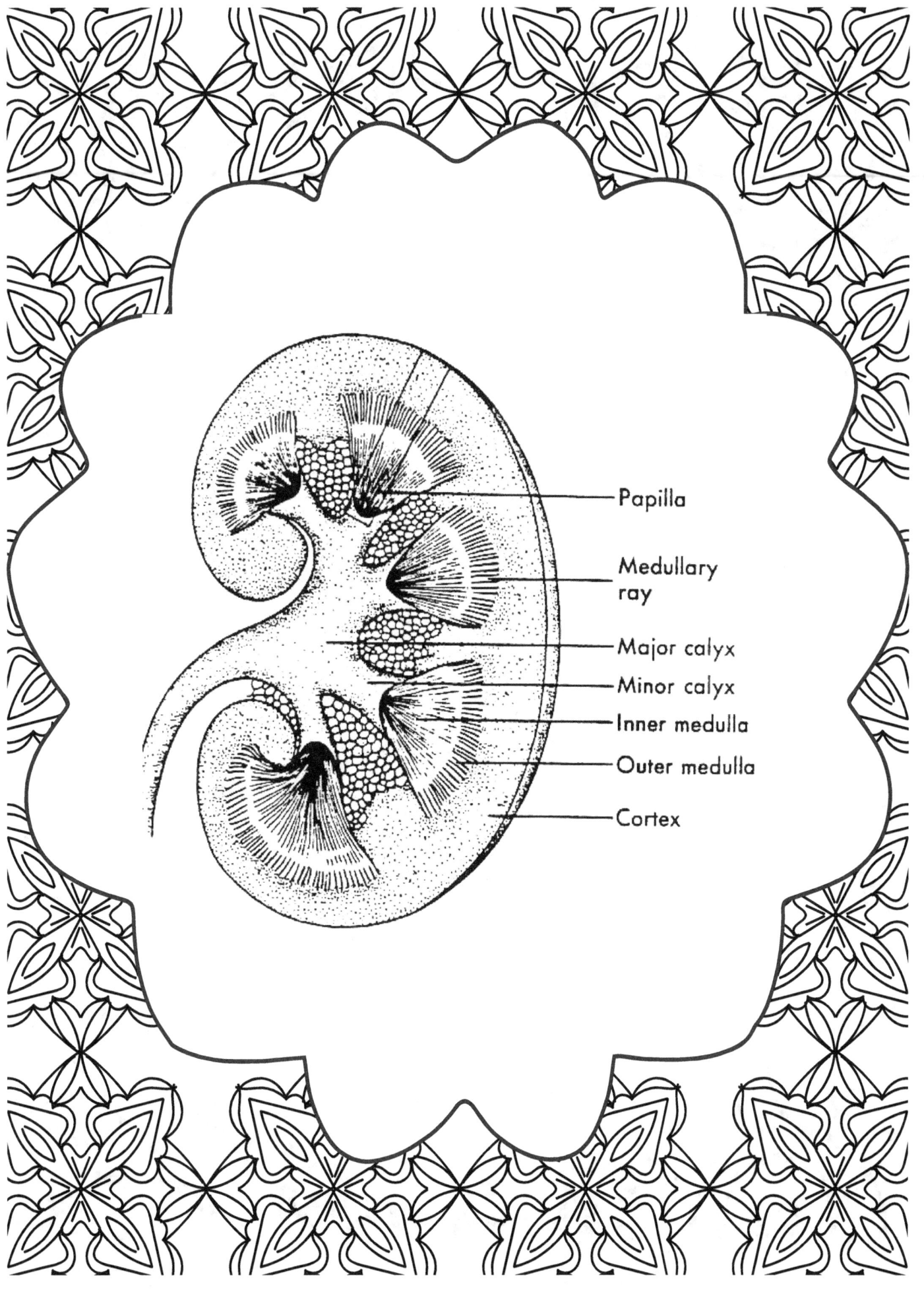

Papilla

Medullary
ray

Major calyx

Minor calyx

Inner medulla

Outer medulla

Cortex

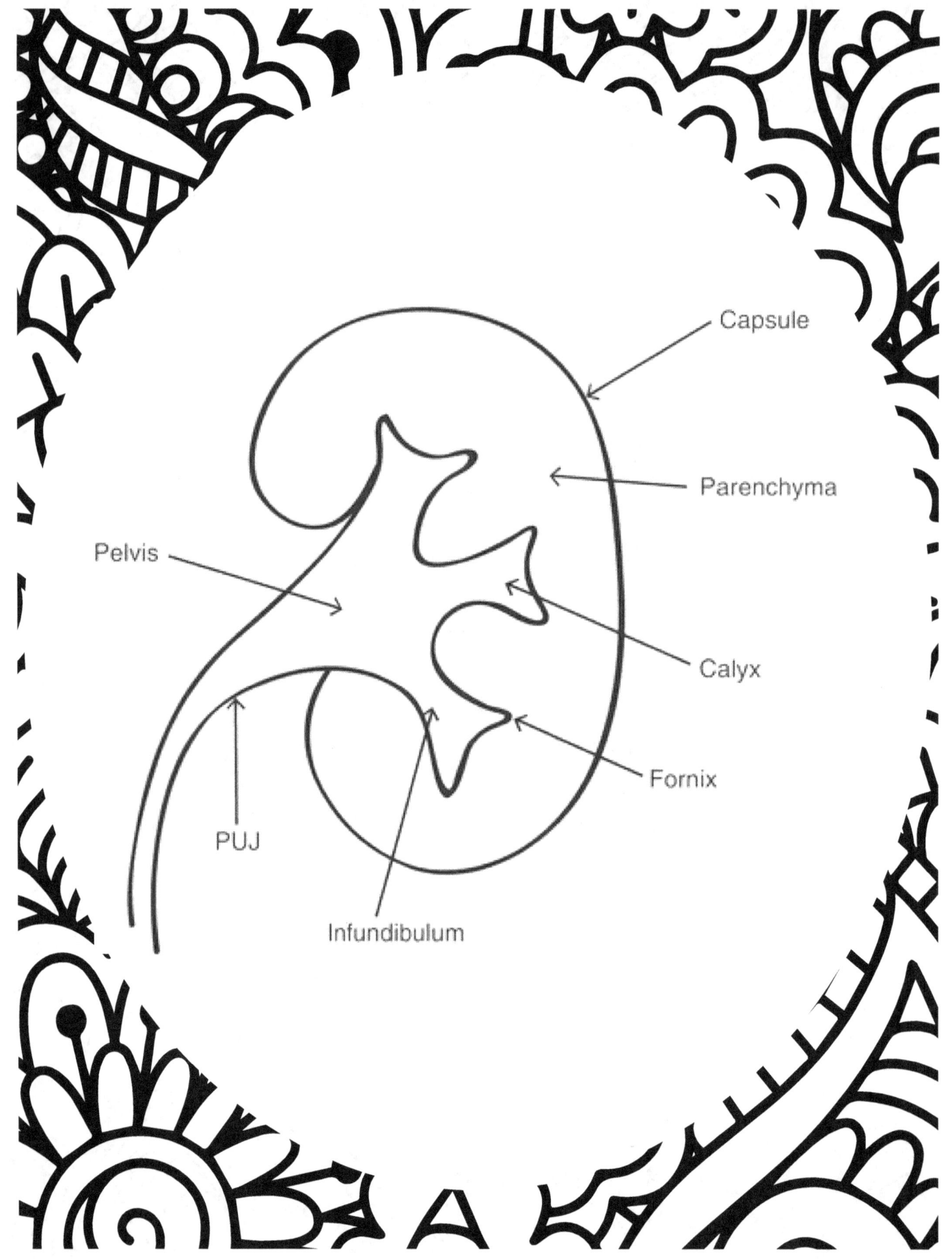

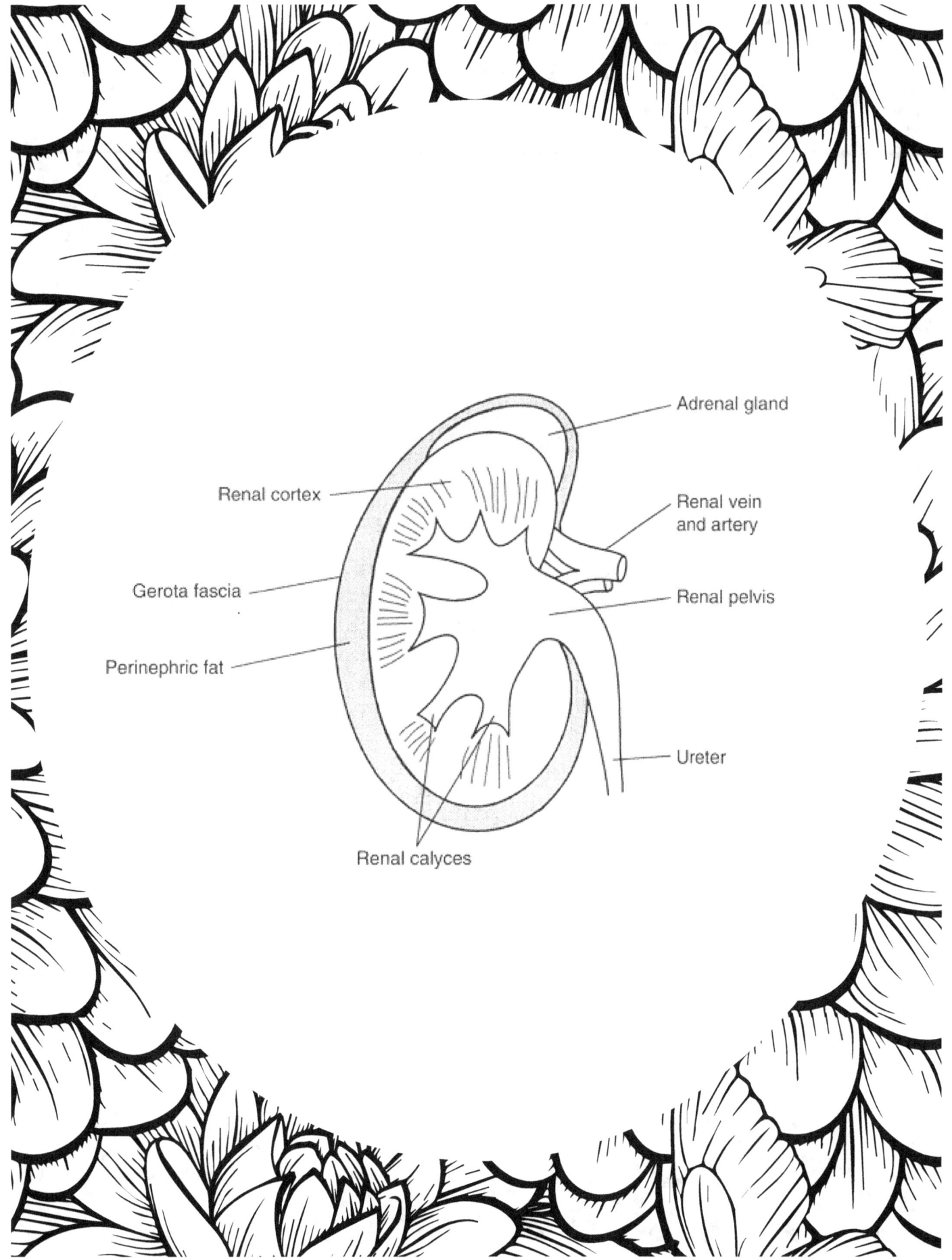

Adrenal gland

Renal cortex

Renal vein
and artery

Gerota fascia

Renal pelvis

Perinephric fat

Ureter

Renal calyces

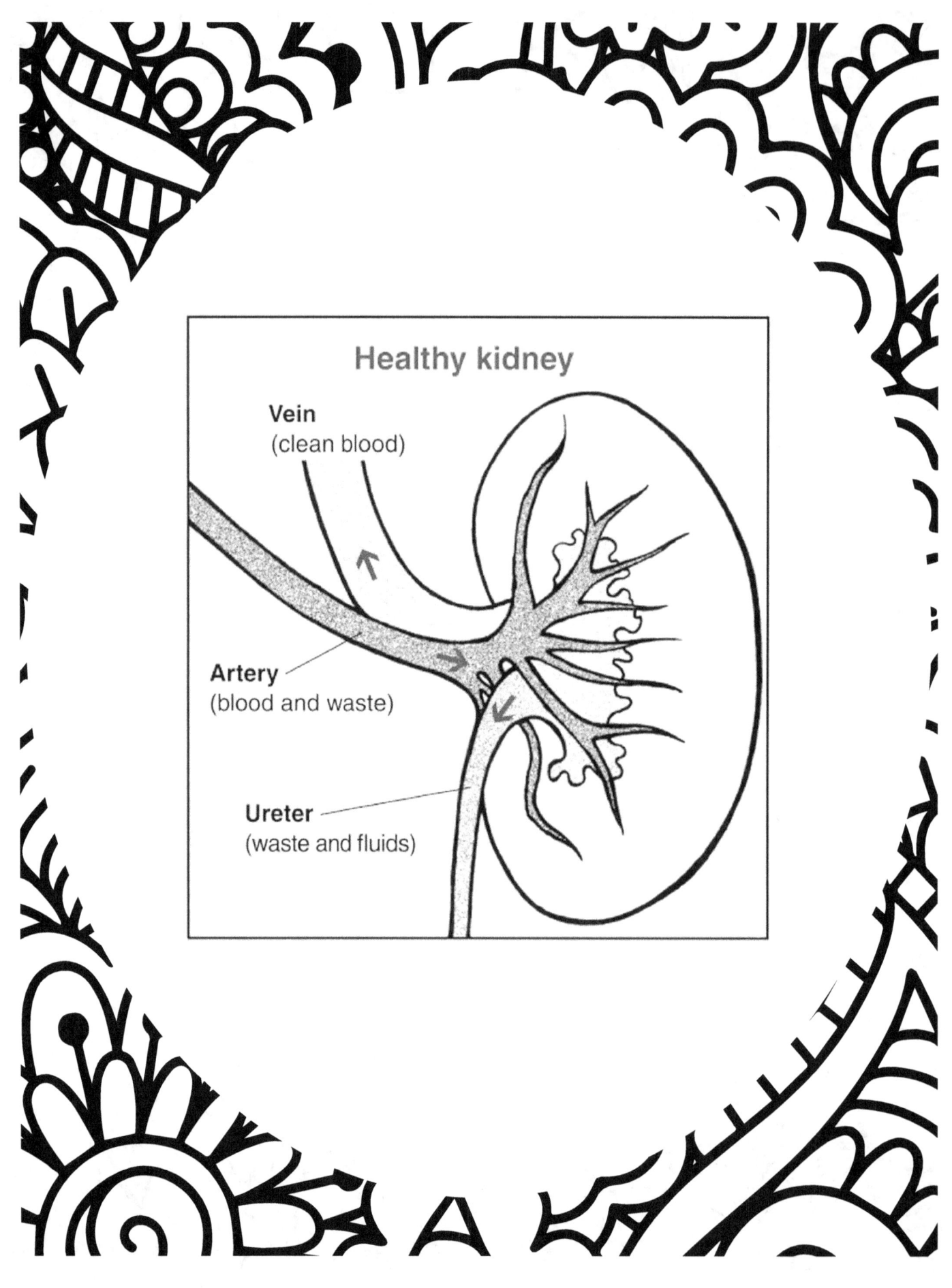

Healthy kidney

Vein
(clean blood)

Artery
(blood and waste)

Ureter
(waste and fluids)

Anatomy of Kidney

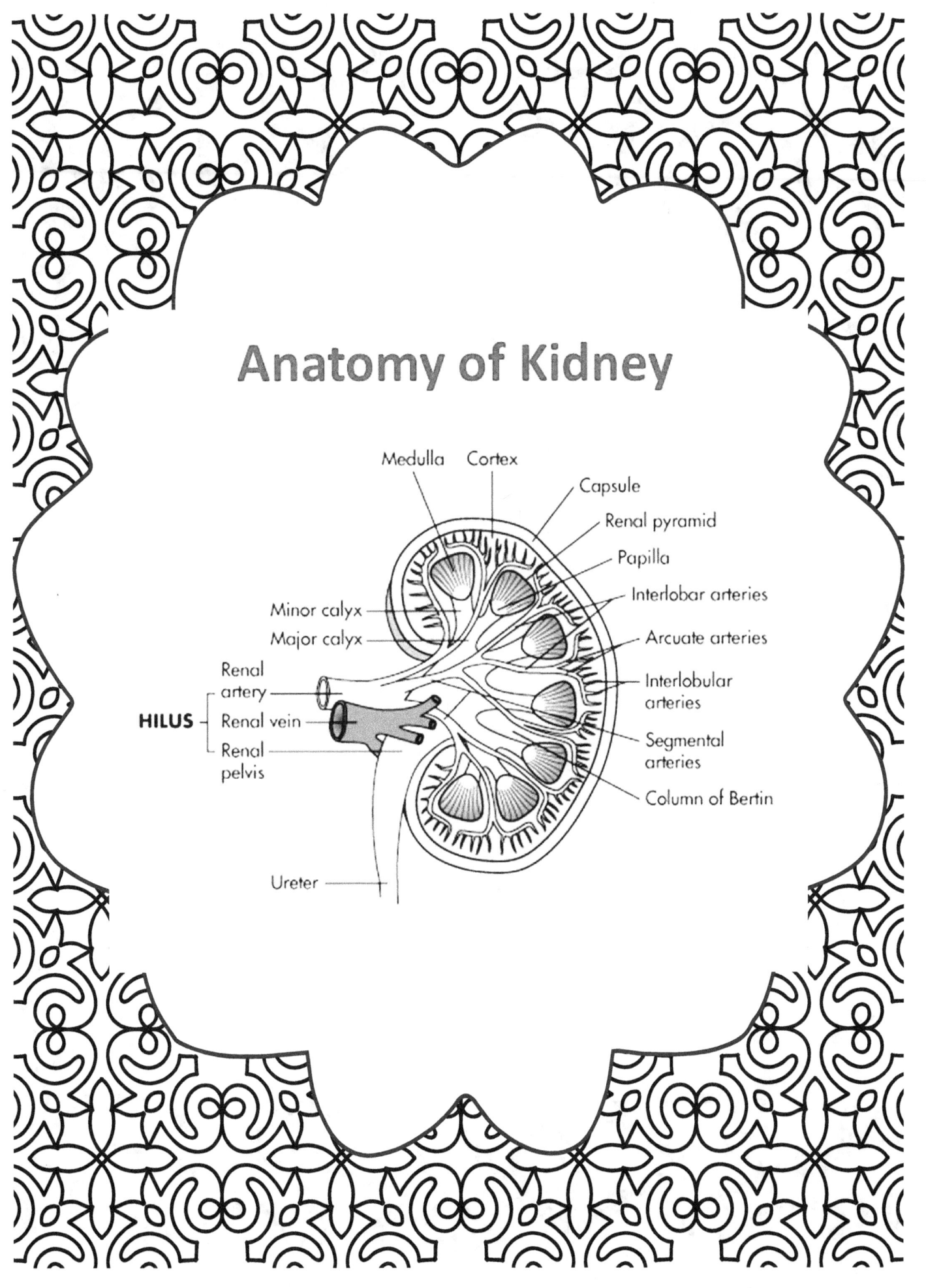

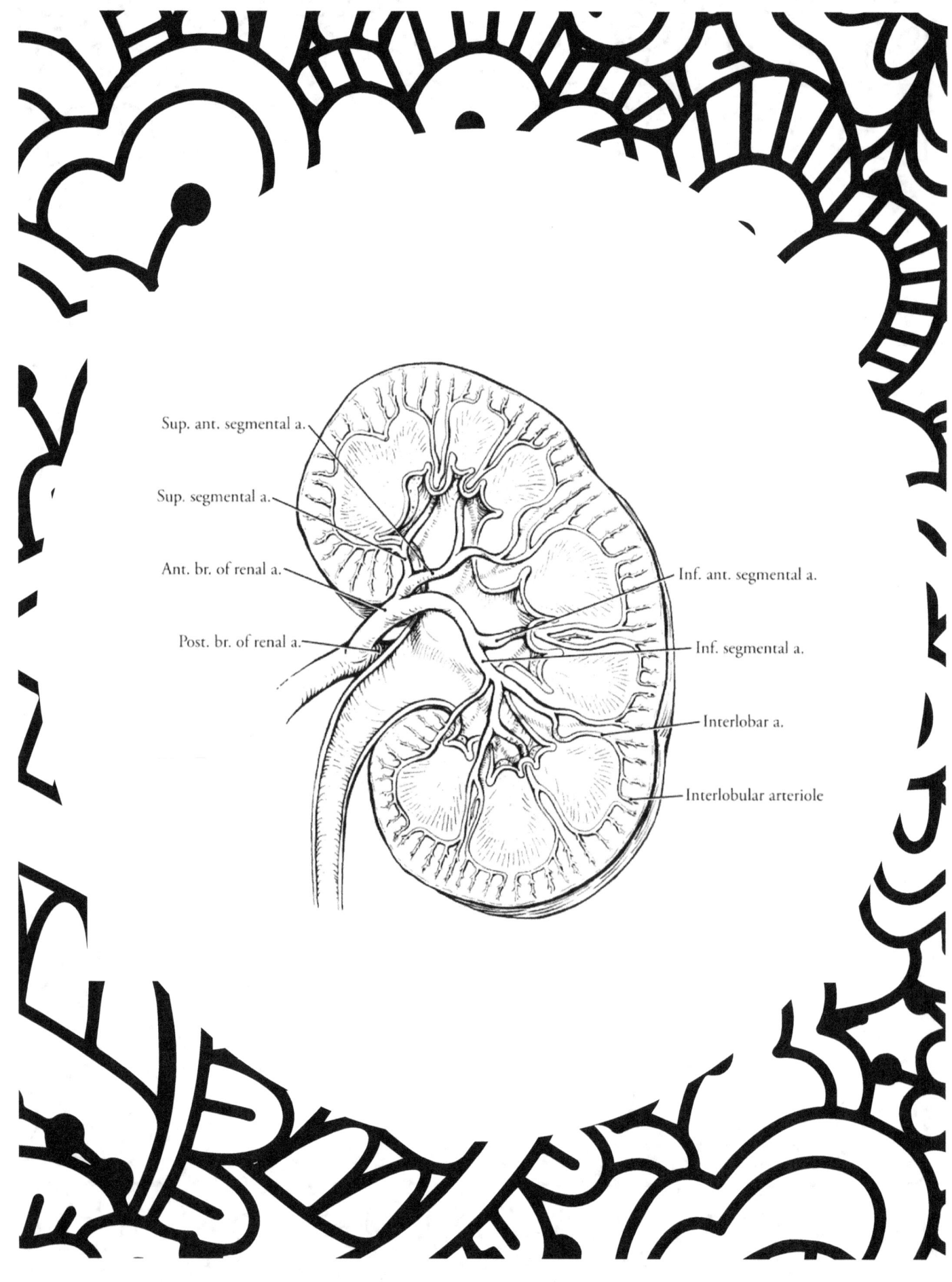

Sup. ant. segmental a.

Sup. segmental a.

Ant. br. of renal a.

Post. br. of renal a.

Inf. ant. segmental a.

Inf. segmental a.

Interlobar a.

Interlobular arteriole

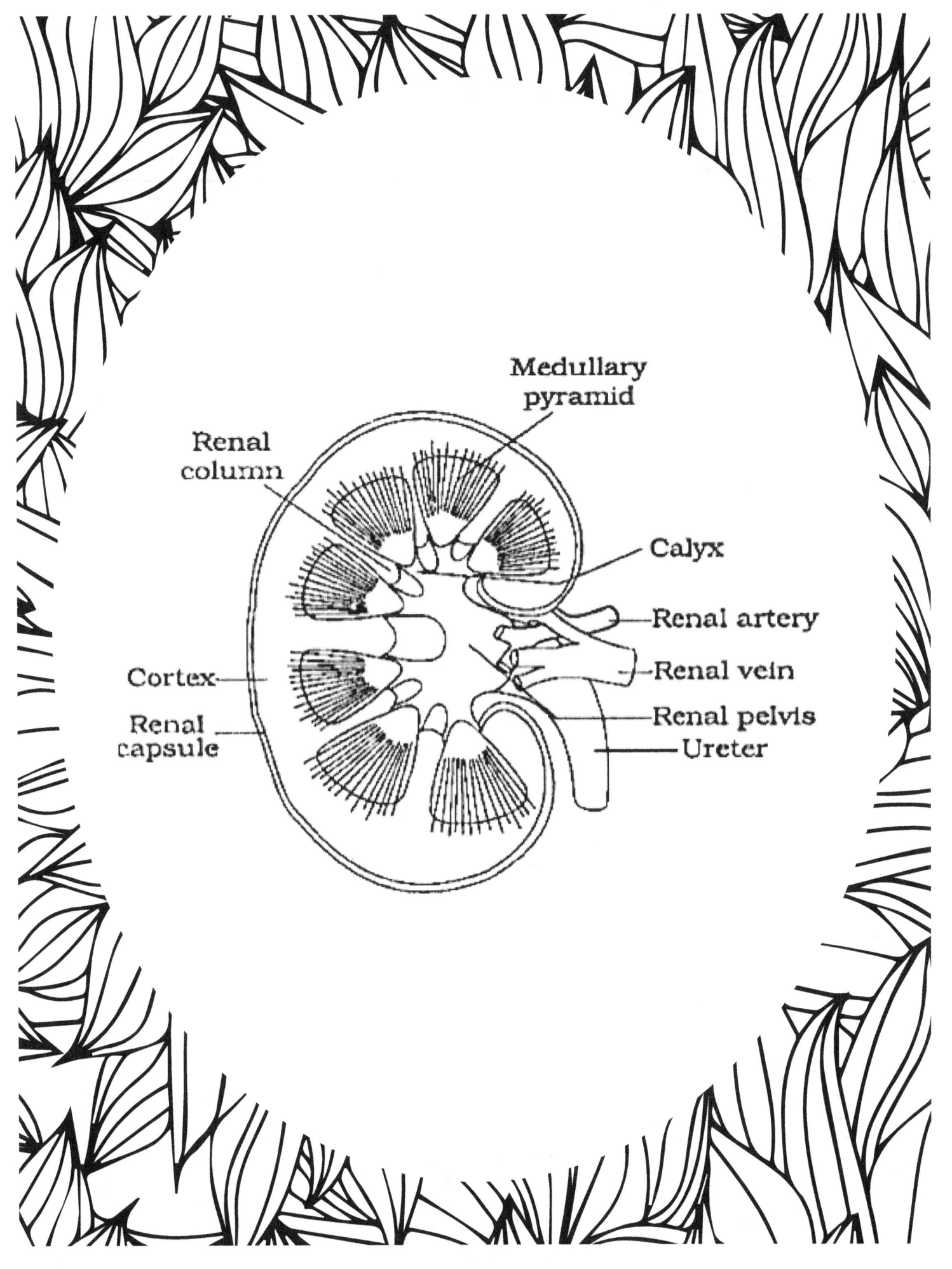

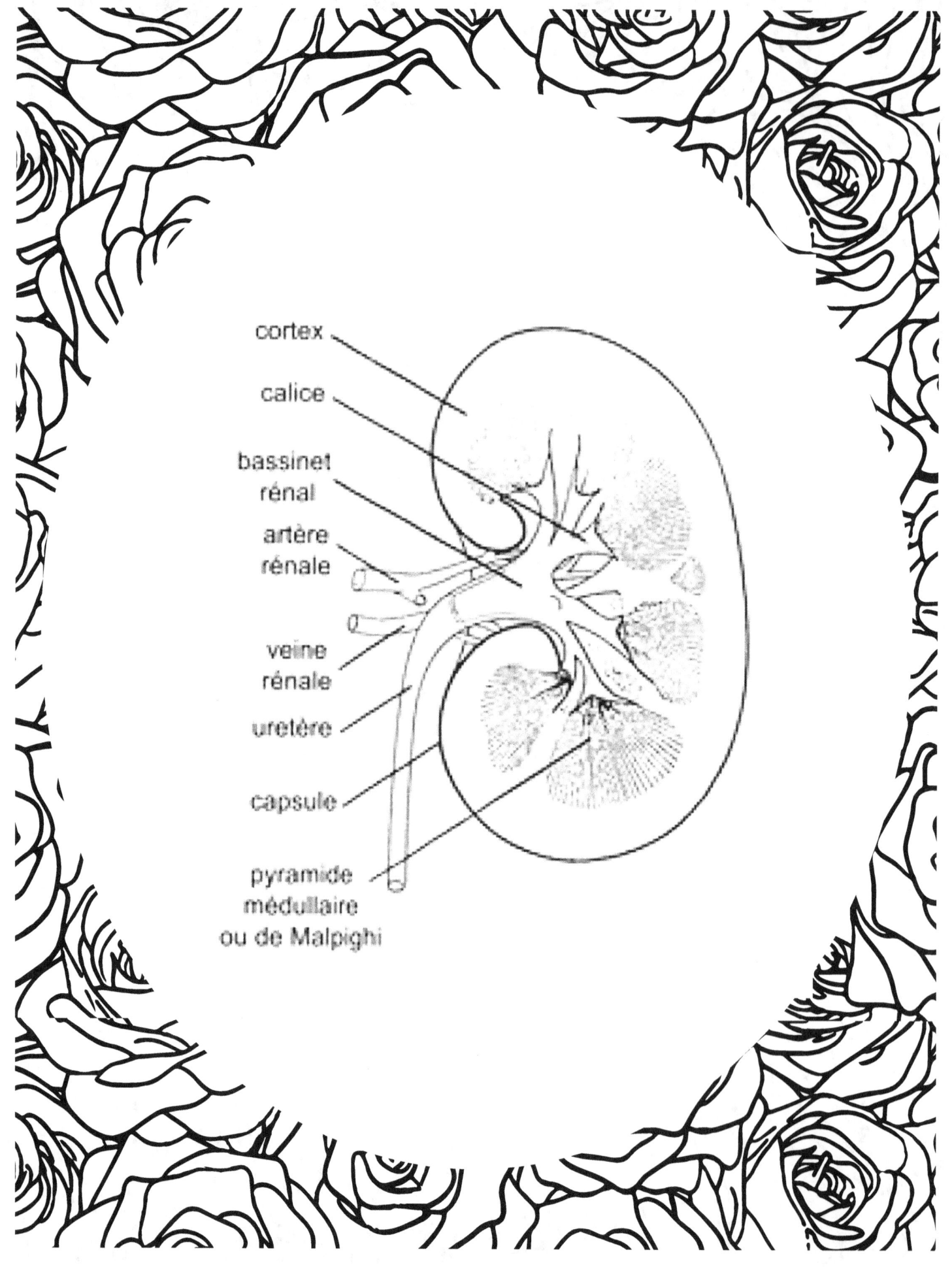

cortex

calice

bassinet
rénal

artère
rénale

veine
rénale

uretère

capsule

pyramide
médullaire
ou de Malpighi

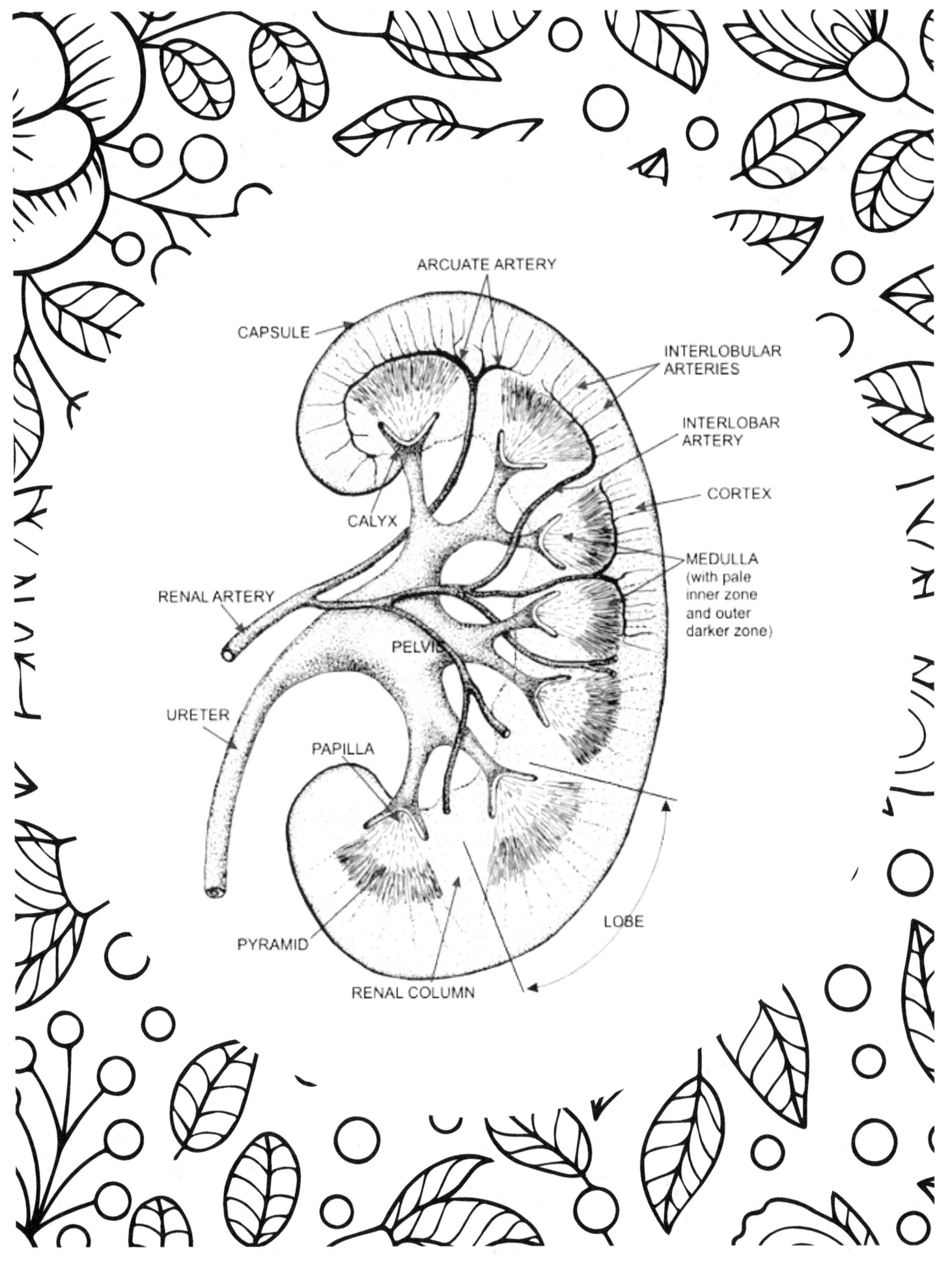

ARCUATE ARTERY

CAPSULE

INTERLOBULAR ARTERIES

INTERLOBAR ARTERY

CORTEX

CALYX

MEDULLA
(with pale inner zone and outer darker zone)

RENAL ARTERY

PELVIS

URETER

PAPILLA

LOBE

PYRAMID

RENAL COLUMN

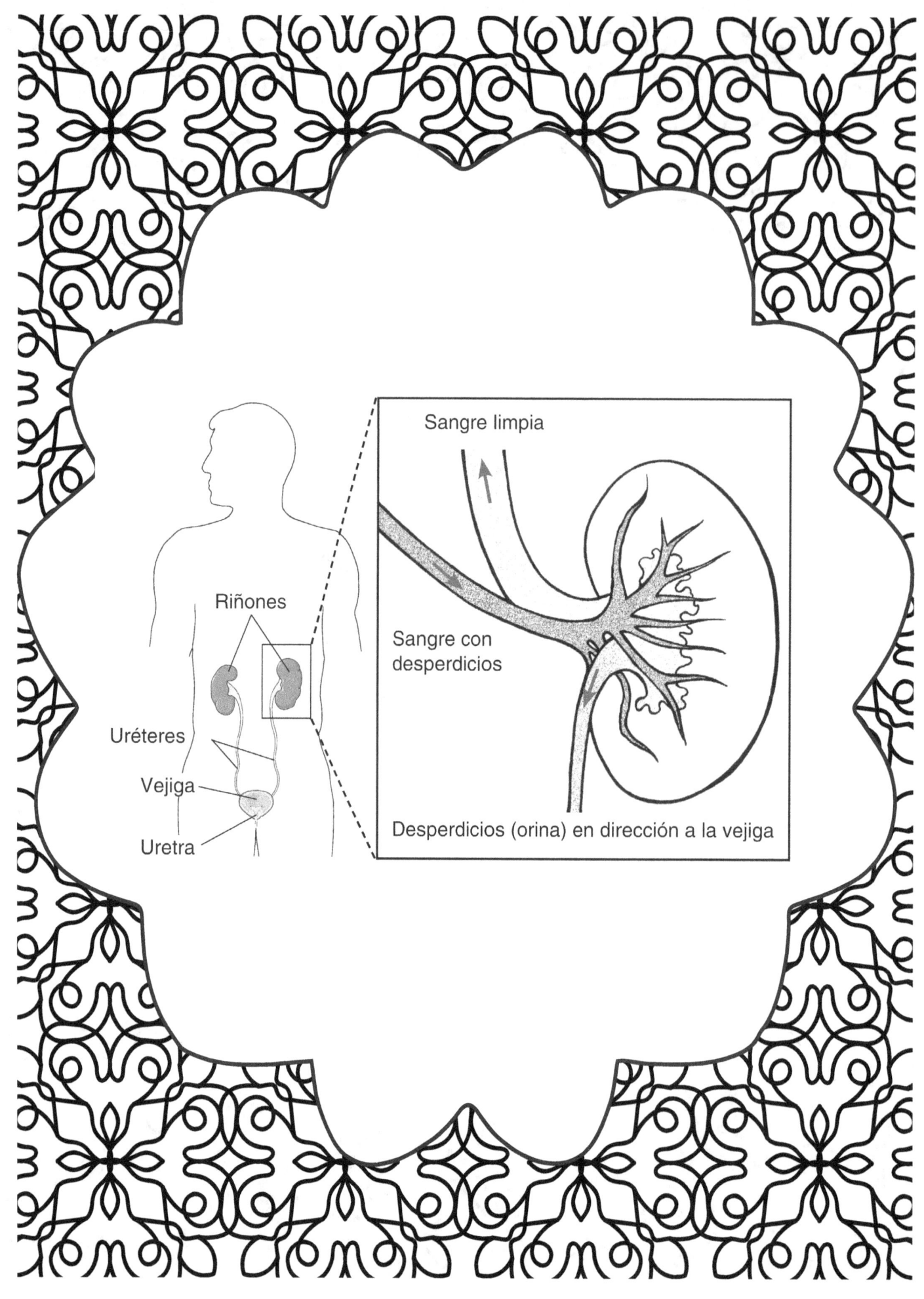

Riñones

Uréteres

Vejiga

Uretra

Sangre limpia

Sangre con
desperdicios

Desperdicios (orina) en dirección a la vejiga

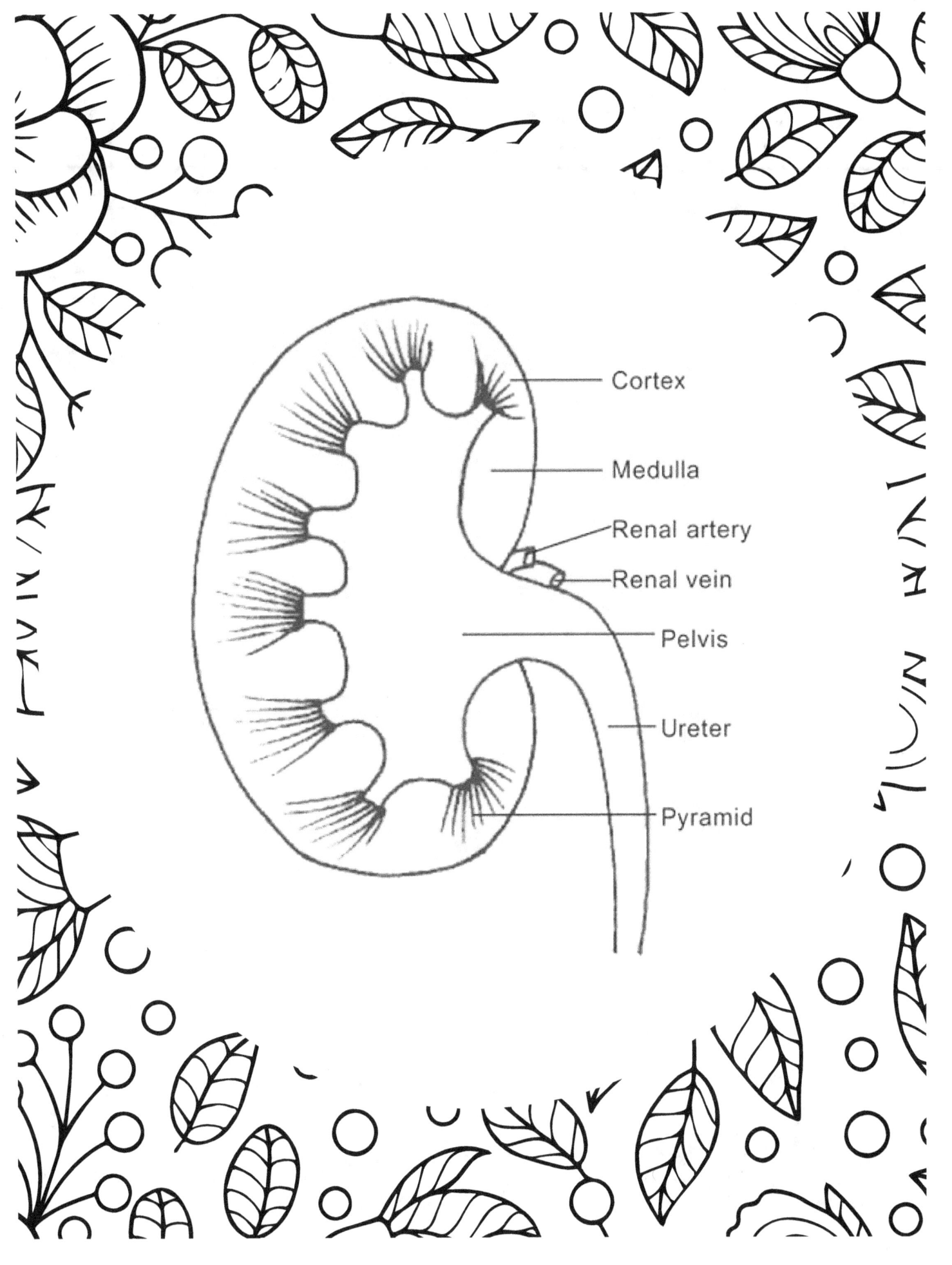

Cortex

Medulla

Renal artery

Renal vein

Pelvis

Ureter

Pyramid

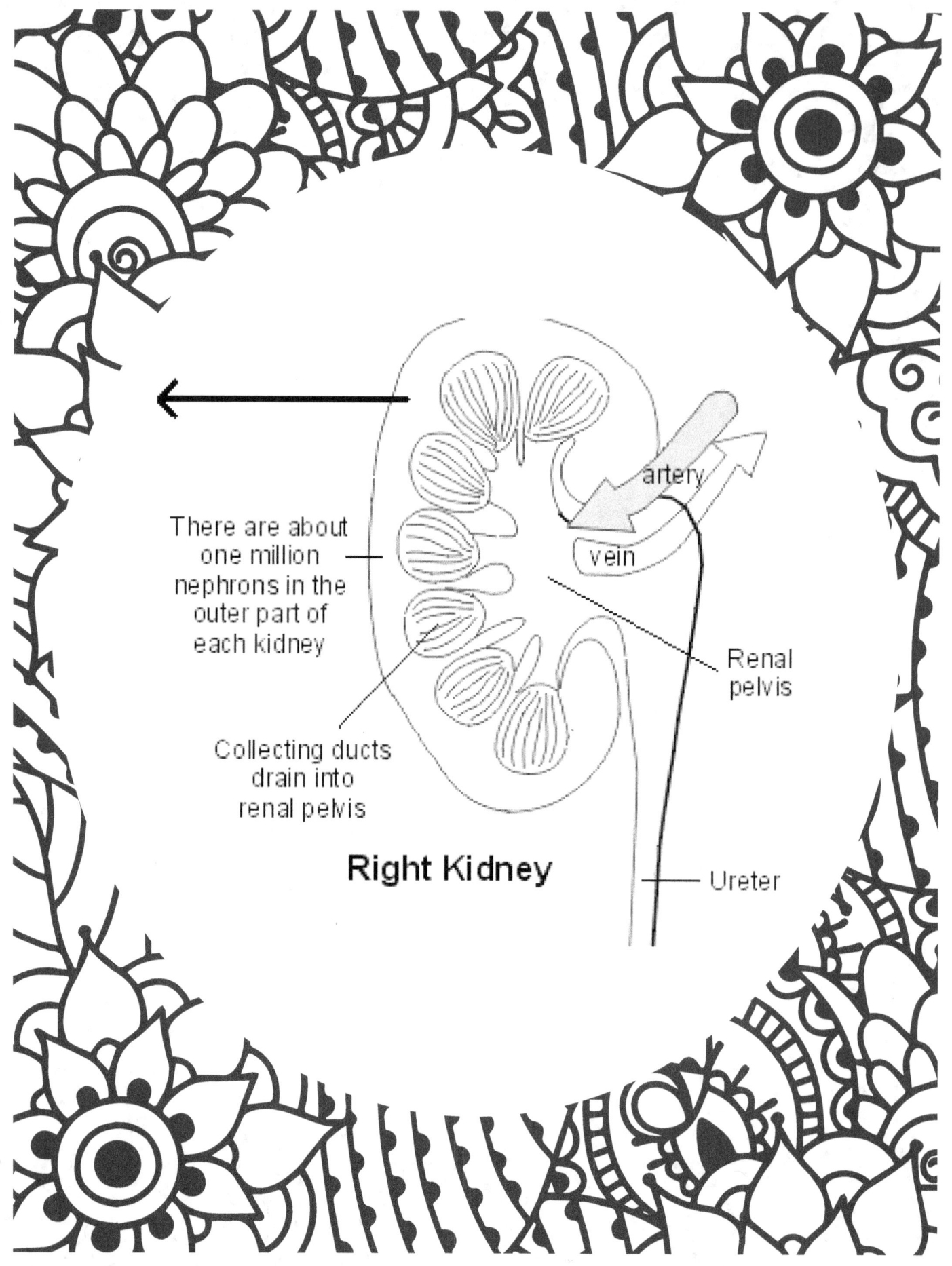

There are about one million nephrons in the outer part of each kidney

Collecting ducts drain into renal pelvis

artery

vein

Renal pelvis

Ureter

Right Kidney

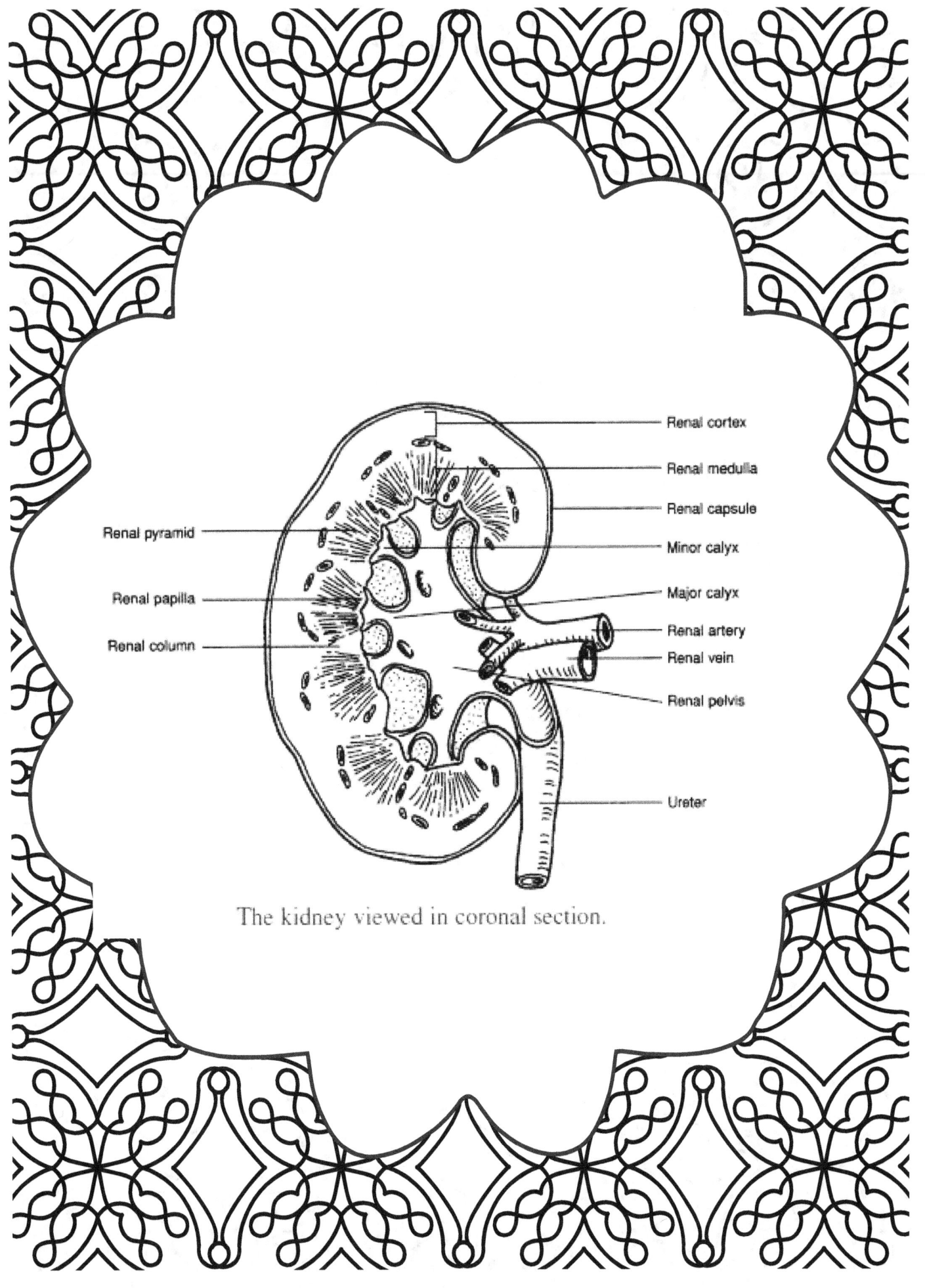

Renal cortex

Renal medulla

Renal capsule

Minor calyx

Major calyx

Renal artery

Renal vein

Renal pelvis

Renal pyramid

Renal papilla

Renal column

Ureter

The kidney viewed in coronal section.

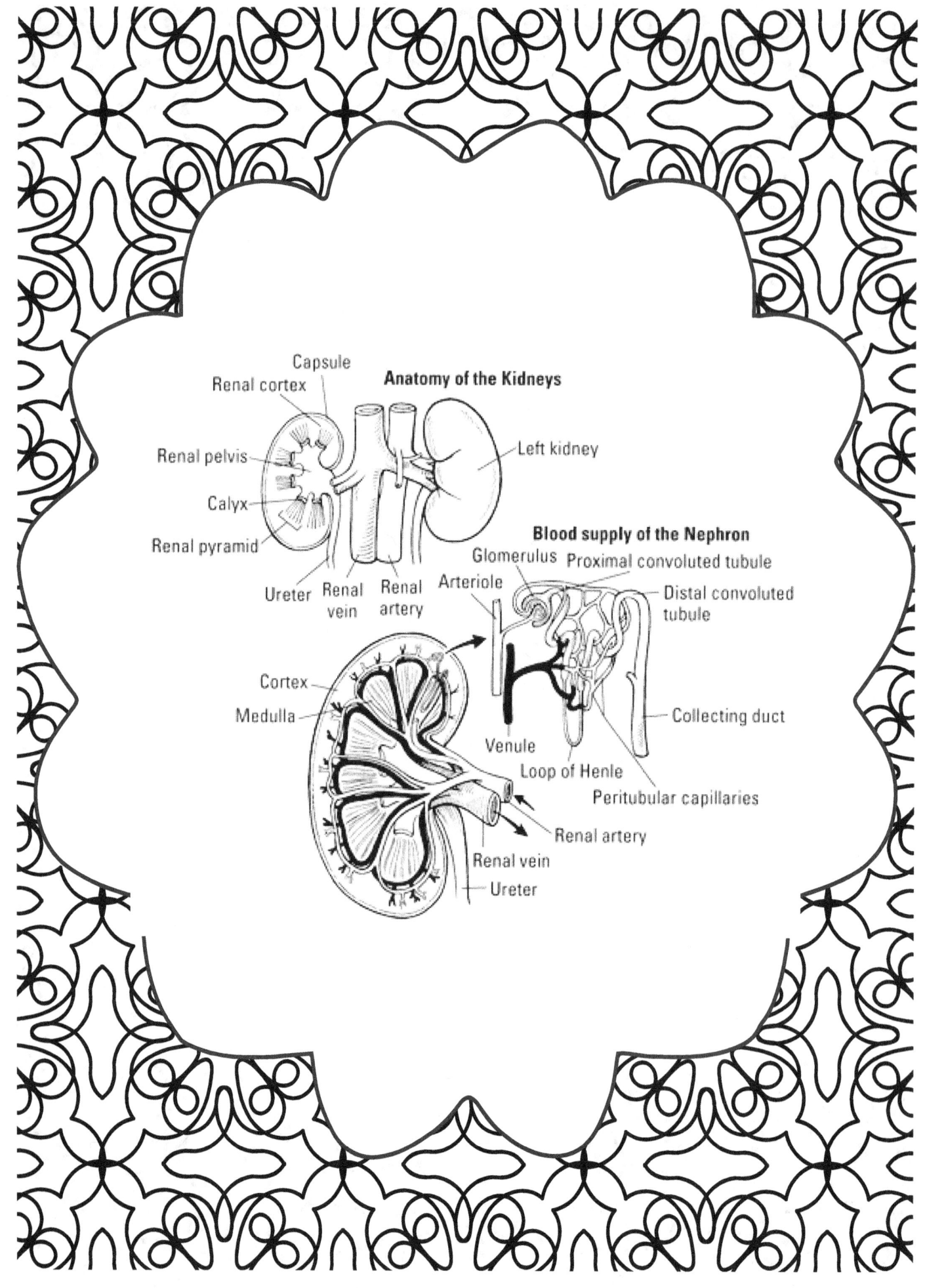

Anatomy of the Kidneys

Capsule
Renal cortex
Renal pelvis
Calyx
Renal pyramid
Ureter
Renal vein
Renal artery
Left kidney

Blood supply of the Nephron

Glomerulus
Proximal convoluted tubule
Arteriole
Distal convoluted tubule
Cortex
Medulla
Venule
Loop of Henle
Collecting duct
Peritubular capillaries
Renal artery
Renal vein
Ureter

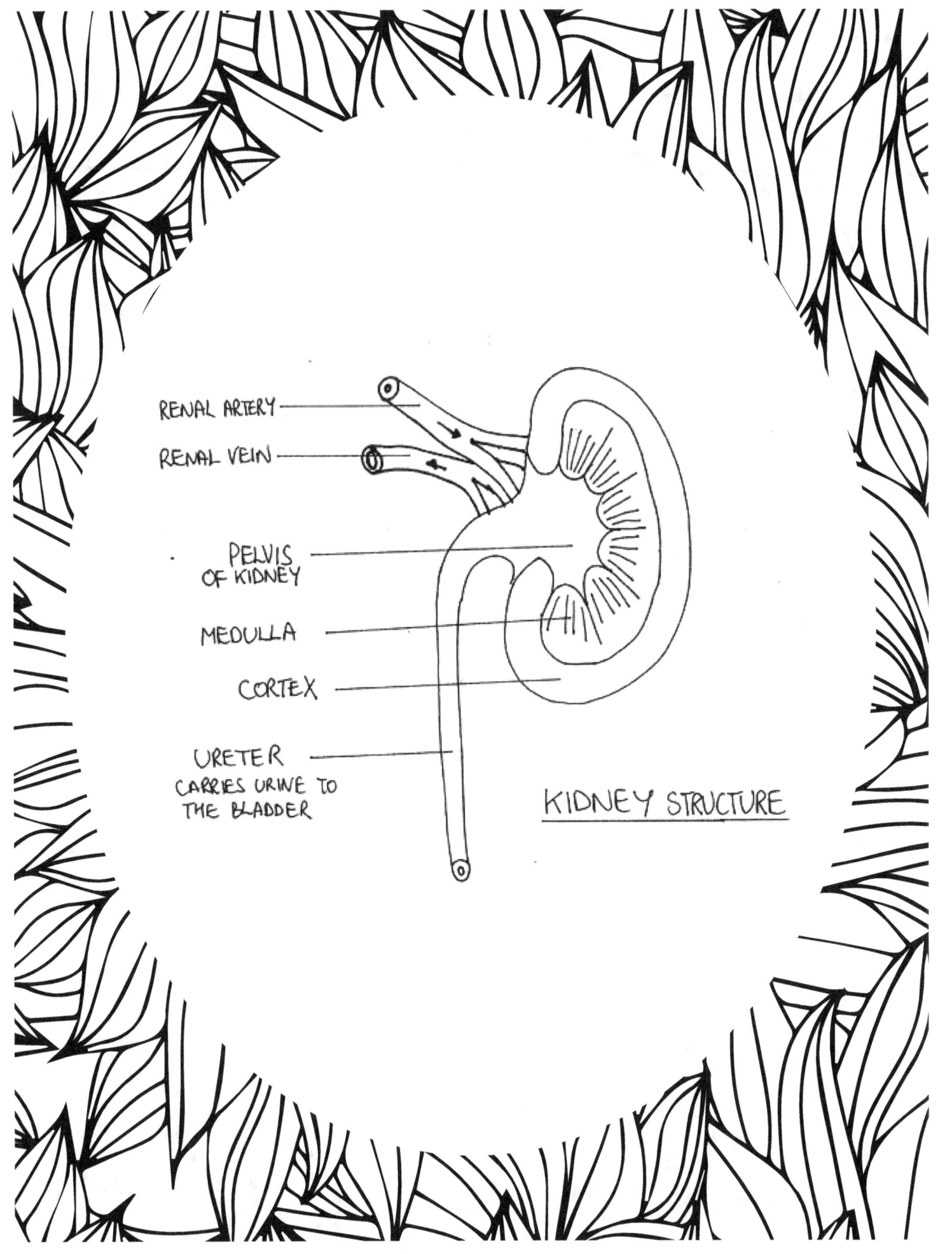

RENAL ARTERY

RENAL VEIN

PELVIS
OF KIDNEY

MEDULLA

CORTEX

URETER
CARRIES URINE TO
THE BLADDER

KIDNEY STRUCTURE

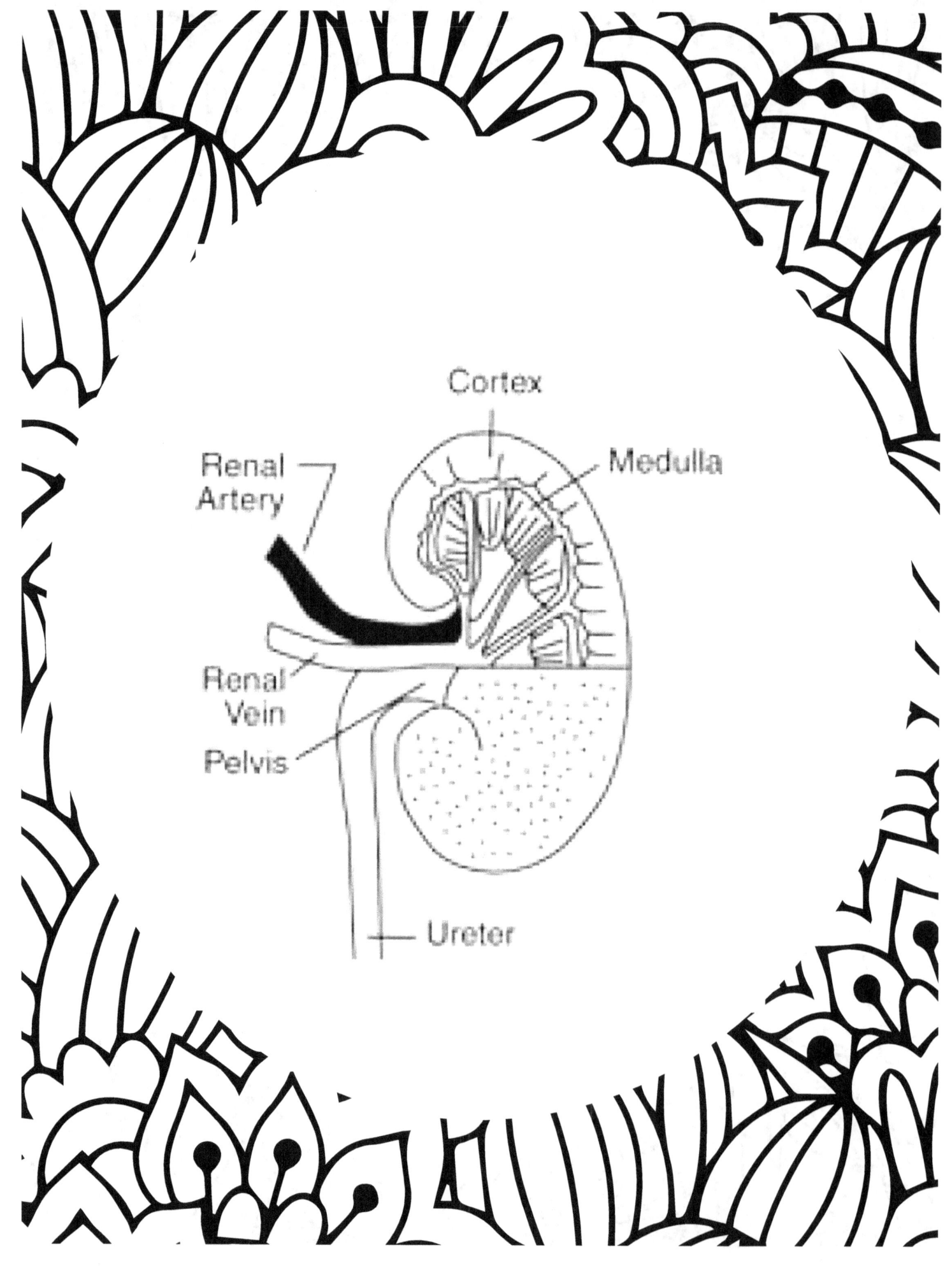

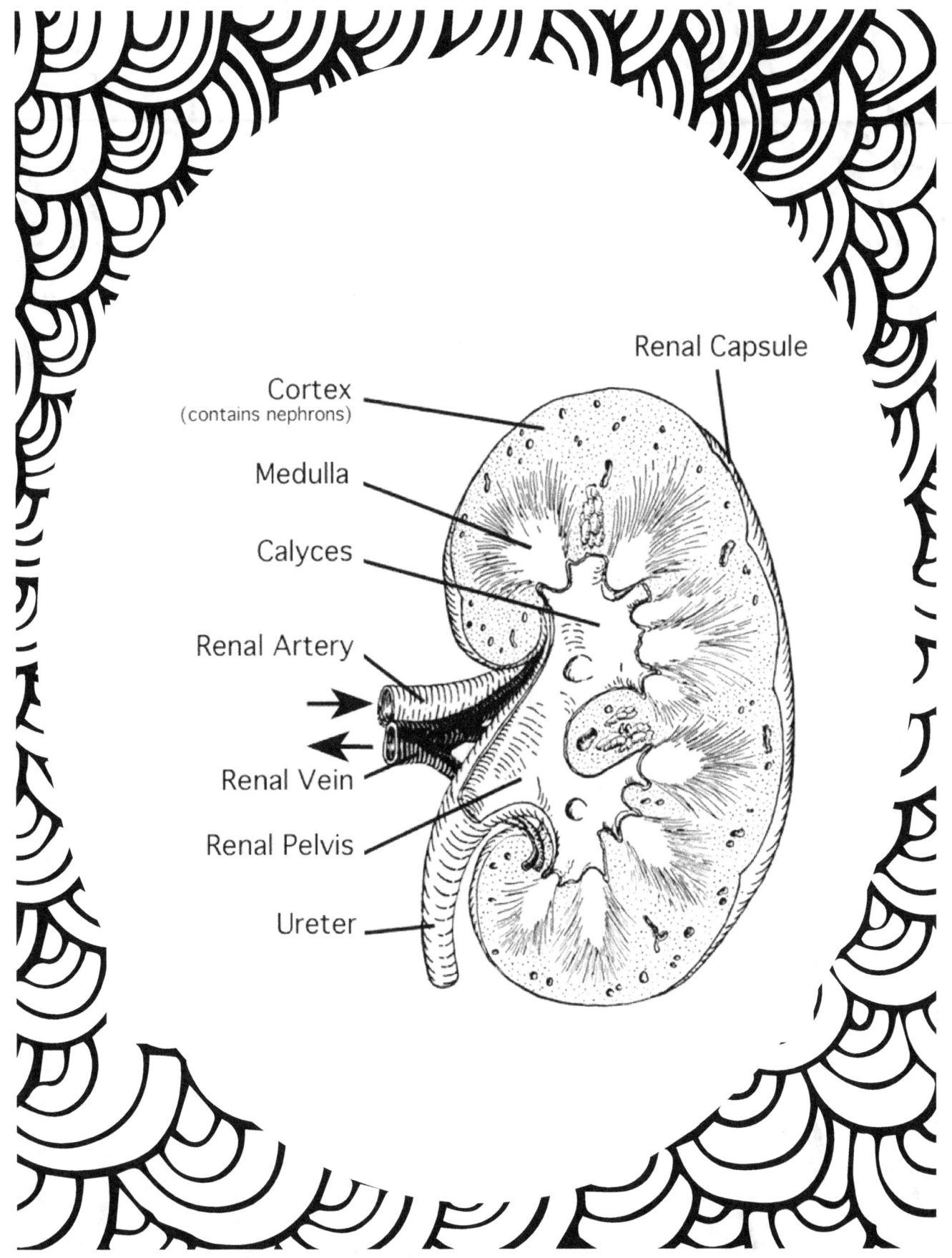

Renal Capsule

Cortex
(contains nephrons)

Medulla

Calyces

Renal Artery

Renal Vein

Renal Pelvis

Ureter

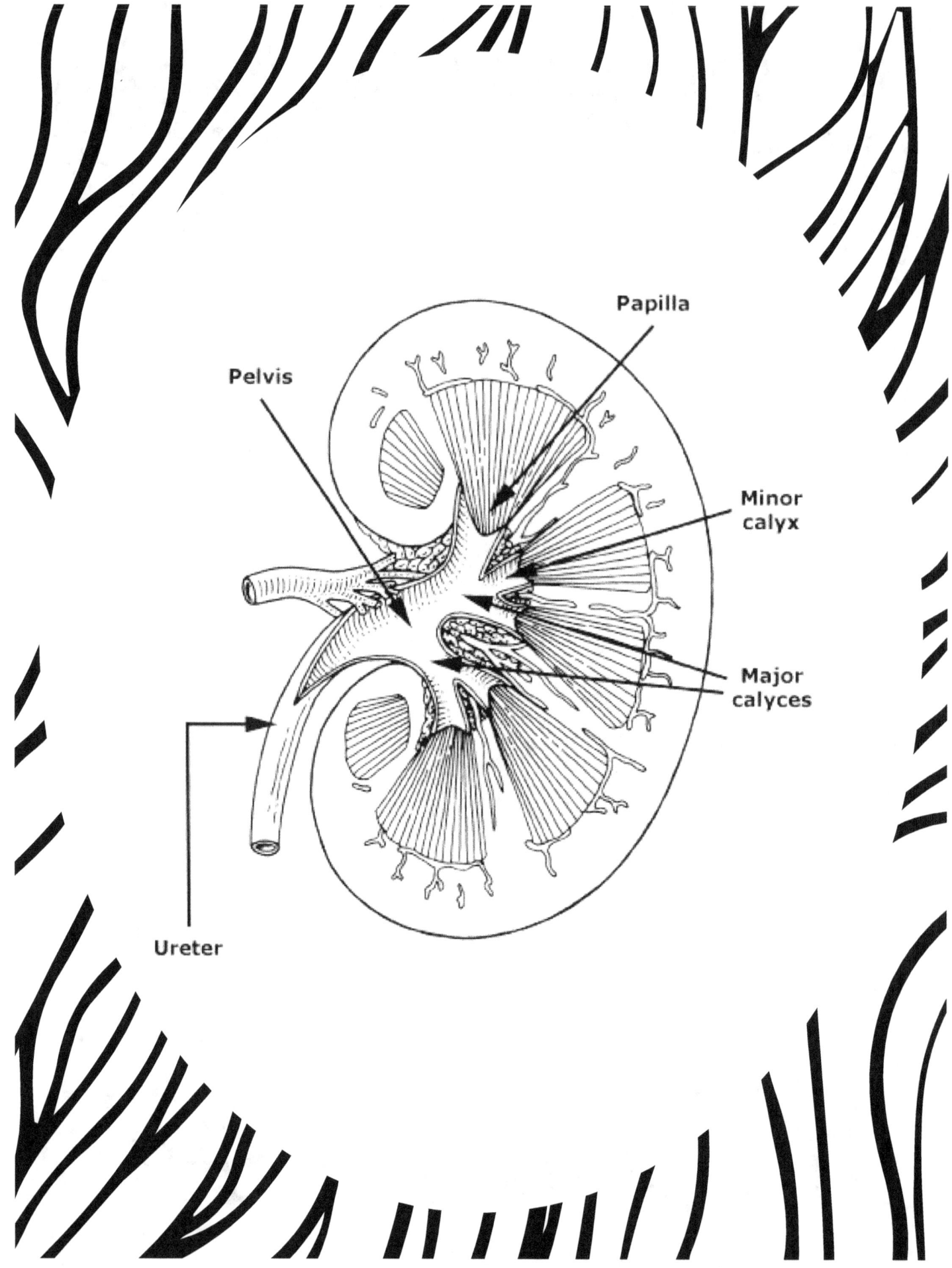

Papilla

Pelvis

Minor
calyx

Major
calyces

Ureter

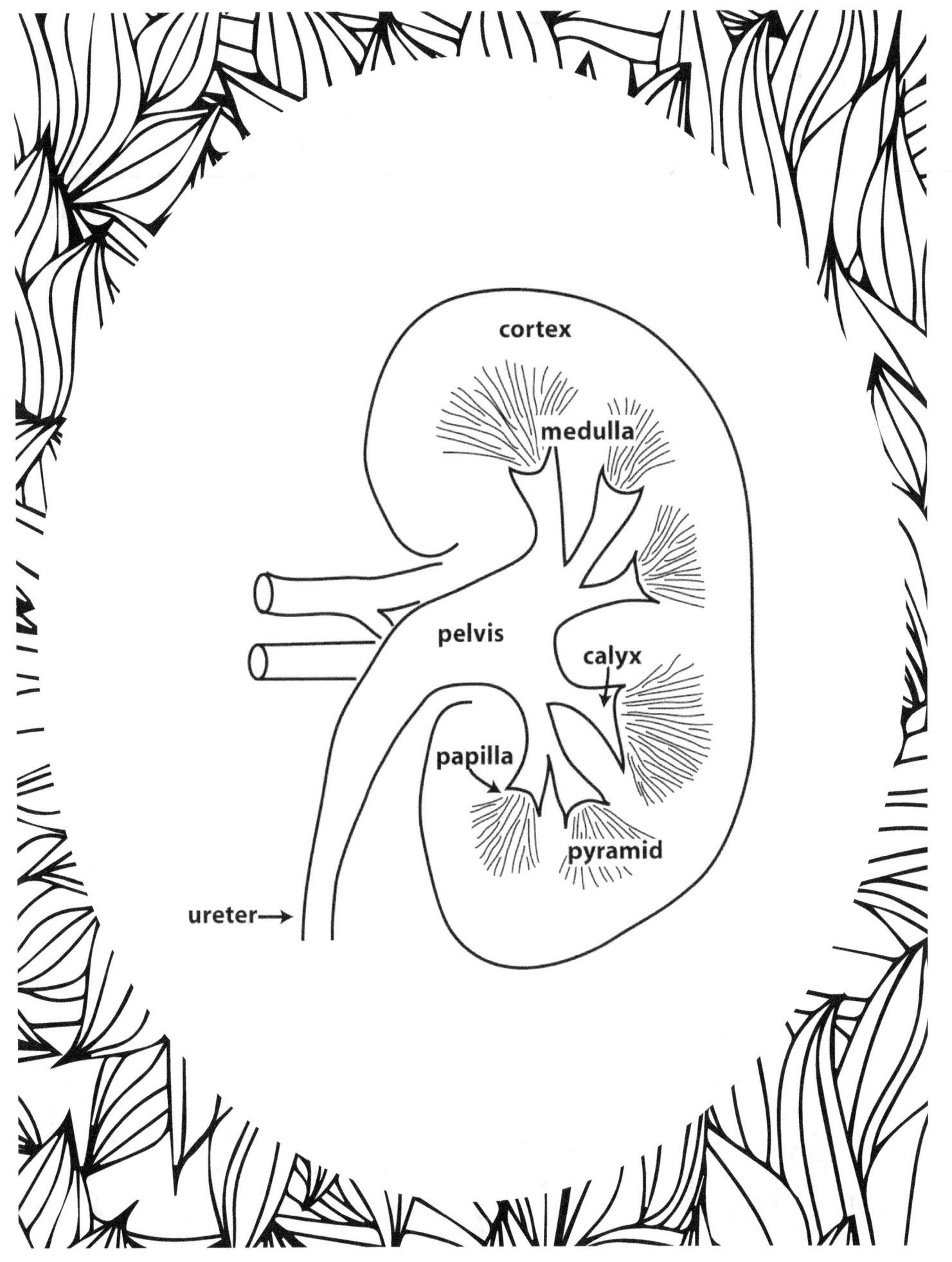

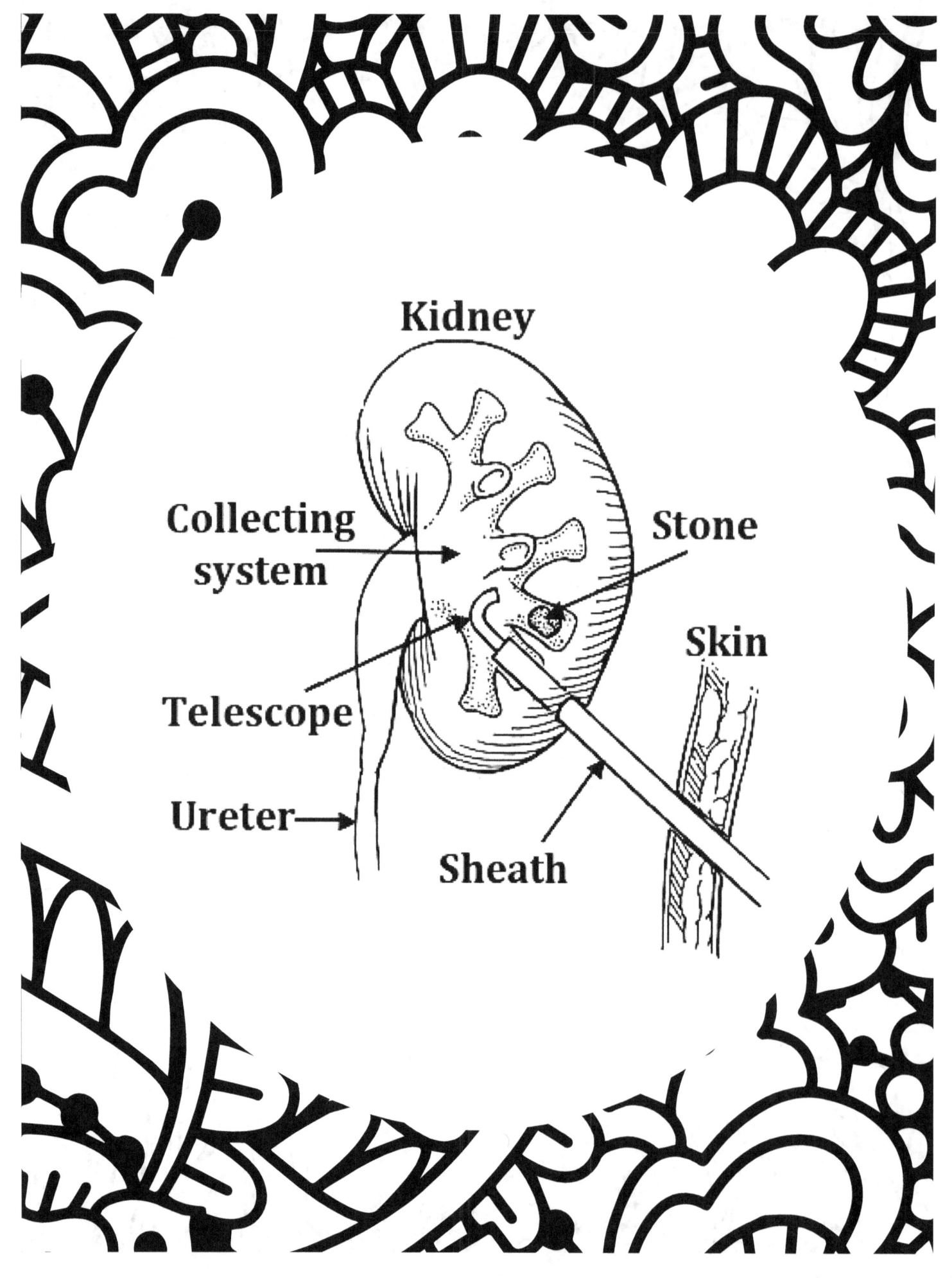

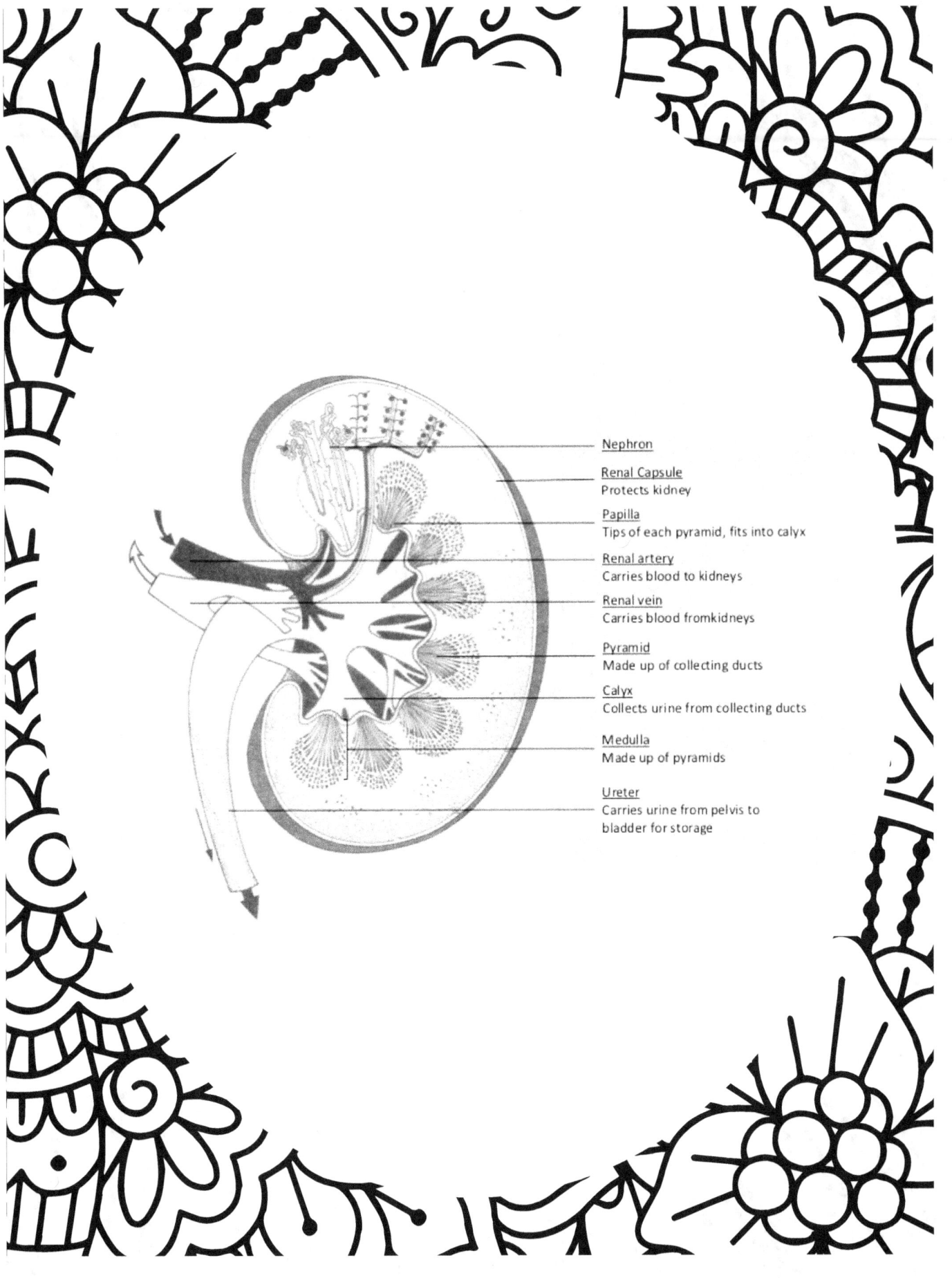

Nephron

Renal Capsule
Protects kidney

Papilla
Tips of each pyramid, fits into calyx

Renal artery
Carries blood to kidneys

Renal vein
Carries blood fromkidneys

Pyramid
Made up of collecting ducts

Calyx
Collects urine from collecting ducts

Medulla
Made up of pyramids

Ureter
Carries urine from pelvis to
bladder for storage

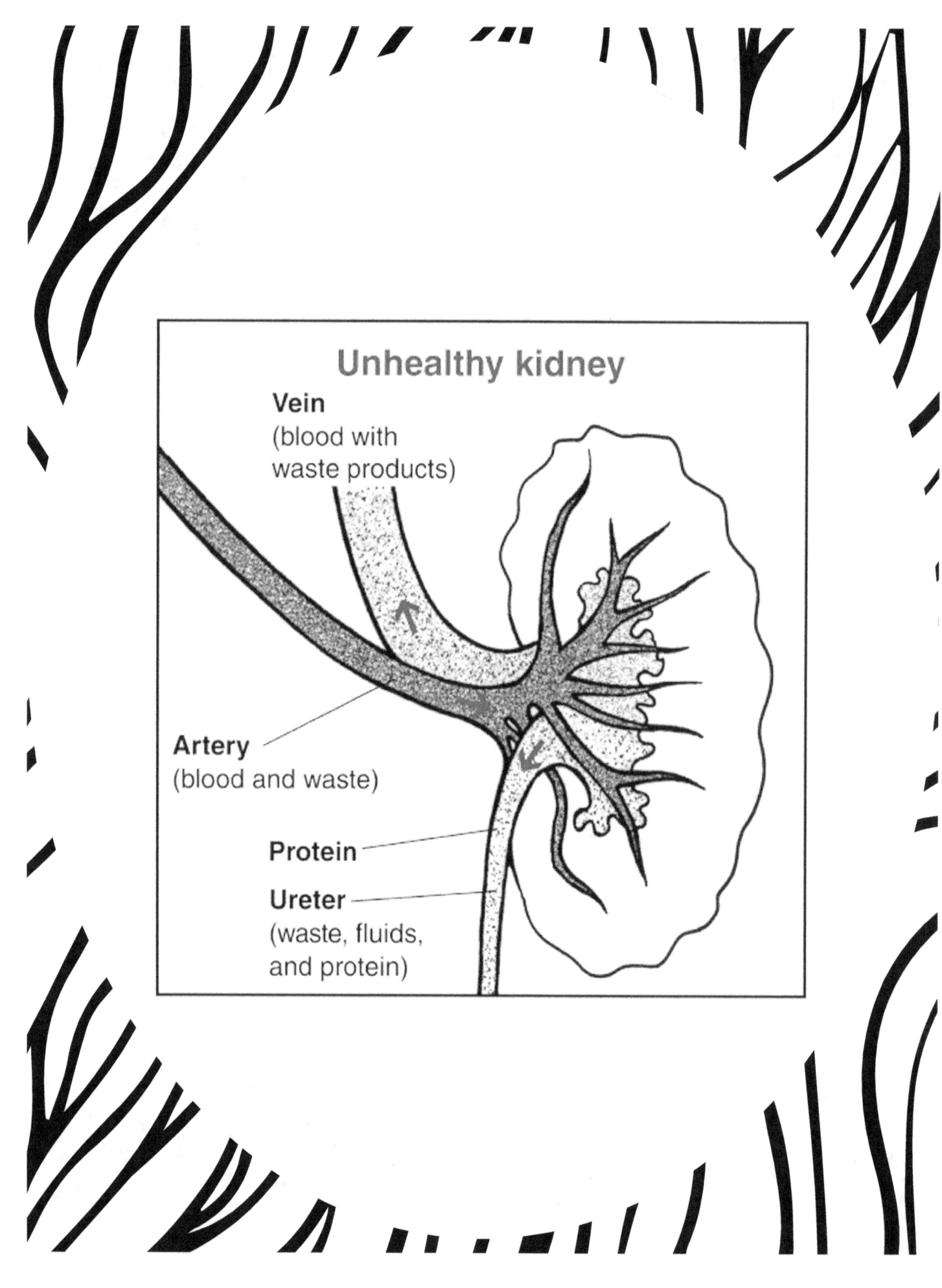

Unhealthy kidney

Vein
(blood with
waste products)

Artery
(blood and waste)

Protein

Ureter
(waste, fluids,
and protein)

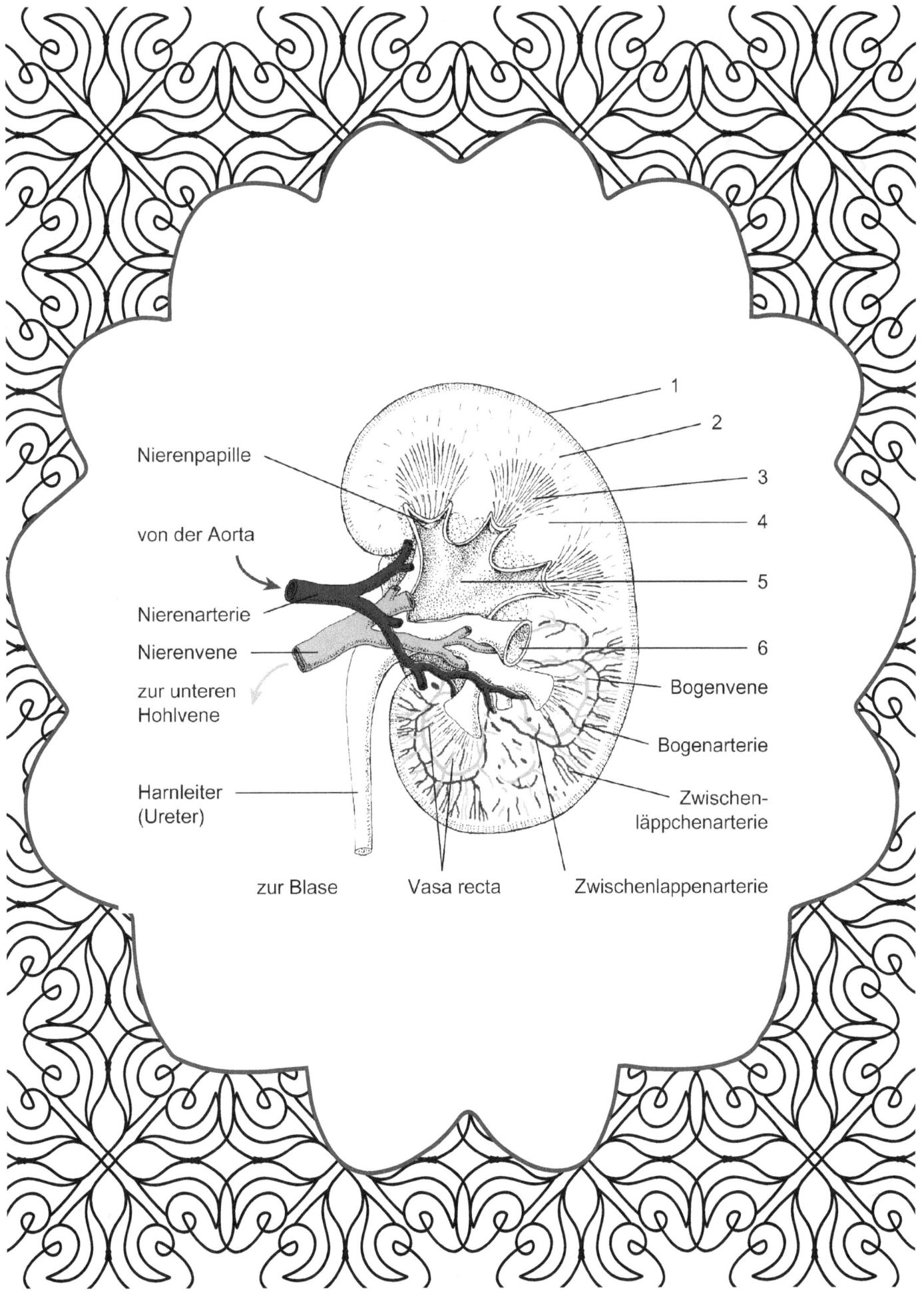

Nierenpapille

von der Aorta

Nierenarterie

Nierenvene

zur unteren
Hohlvene

Harnleiter
(Ureter)

zur Blase

Vasa recta

1
2
3
4
5
6

Bogenvene

Bogenarterie

Zwischen-
läppchenarterie

Zwischenlappenarterie

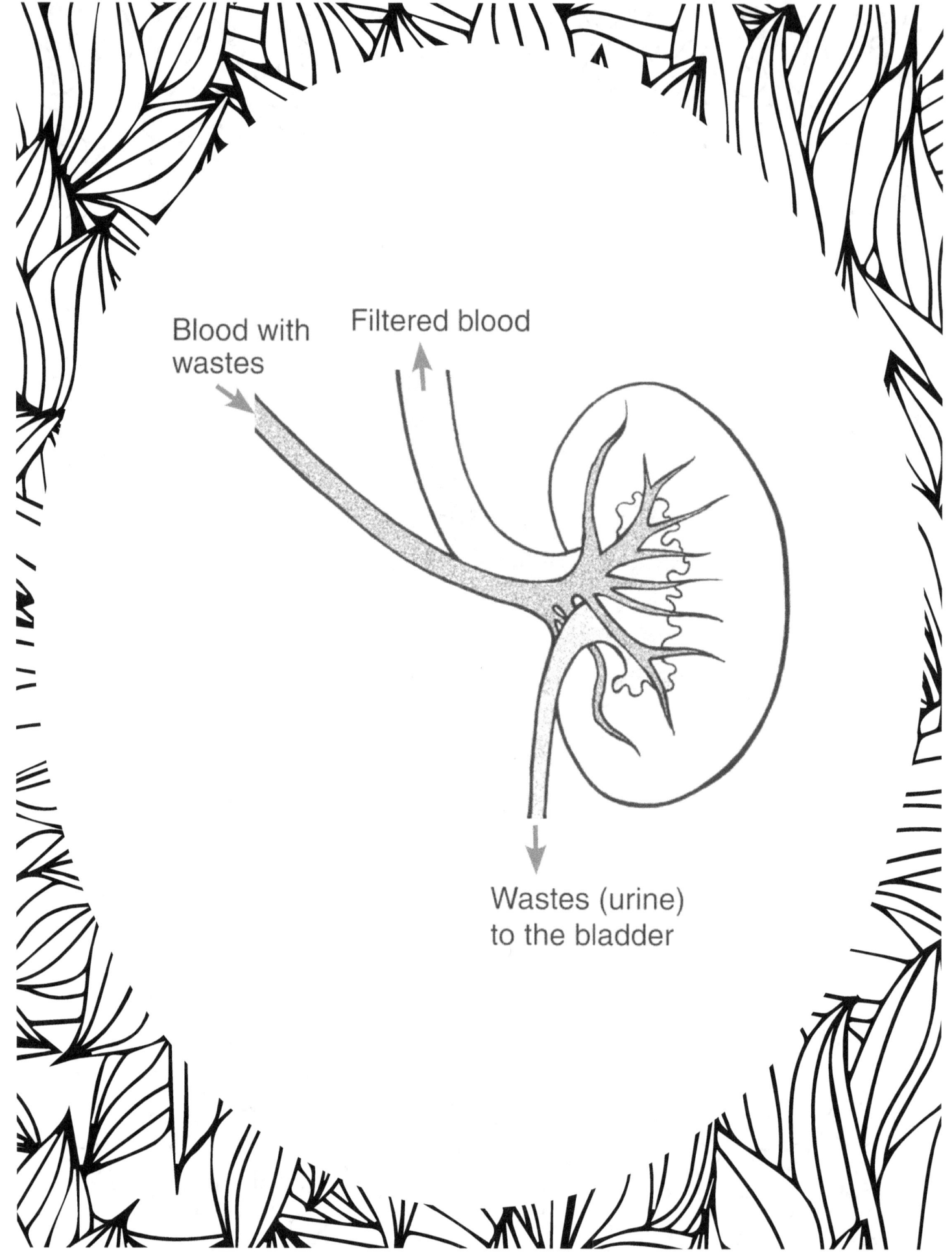

Blood with
wastes

Filtered blood

Wastes (urine)
to the bladder

Kidney Anatomy

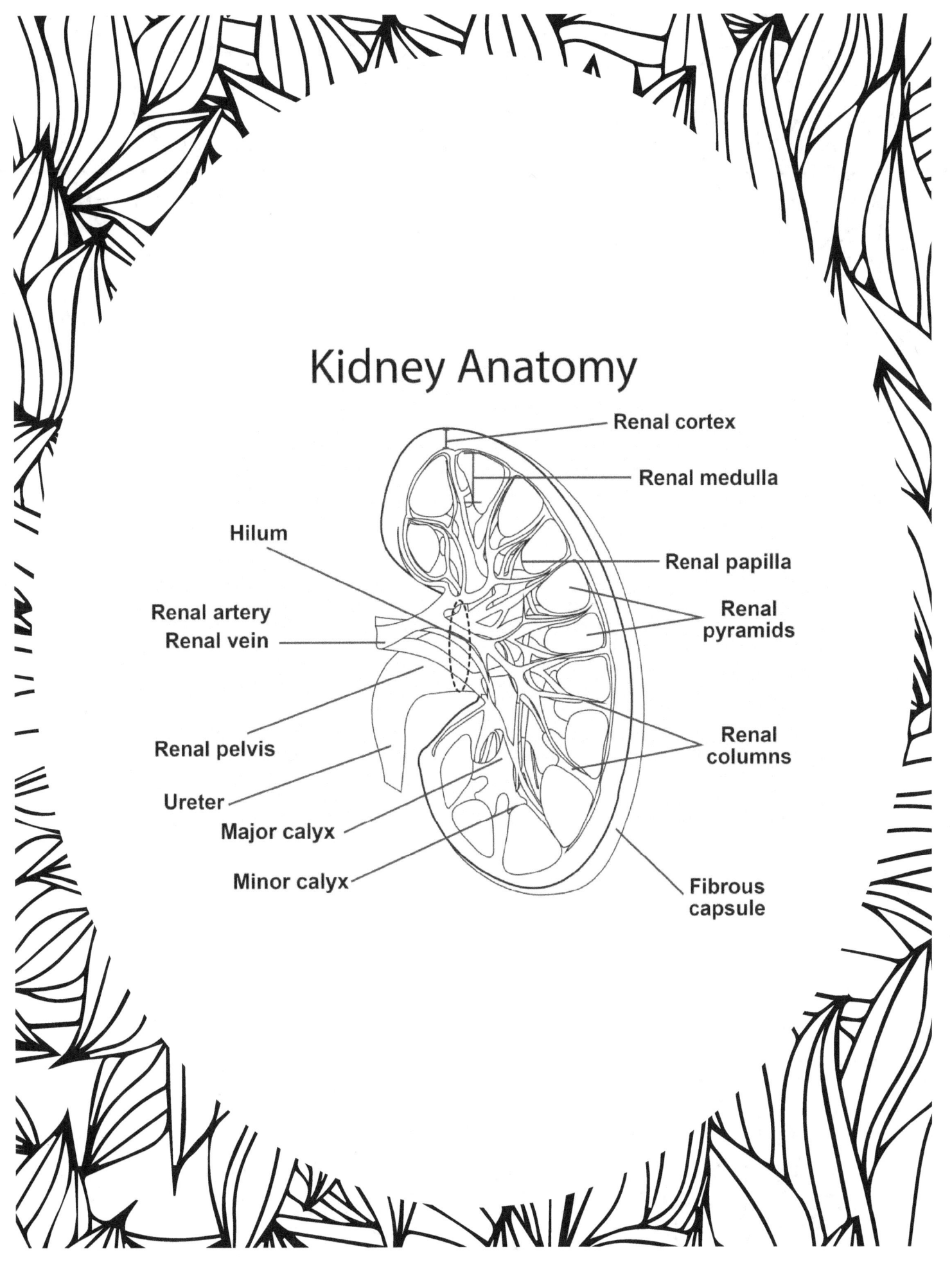

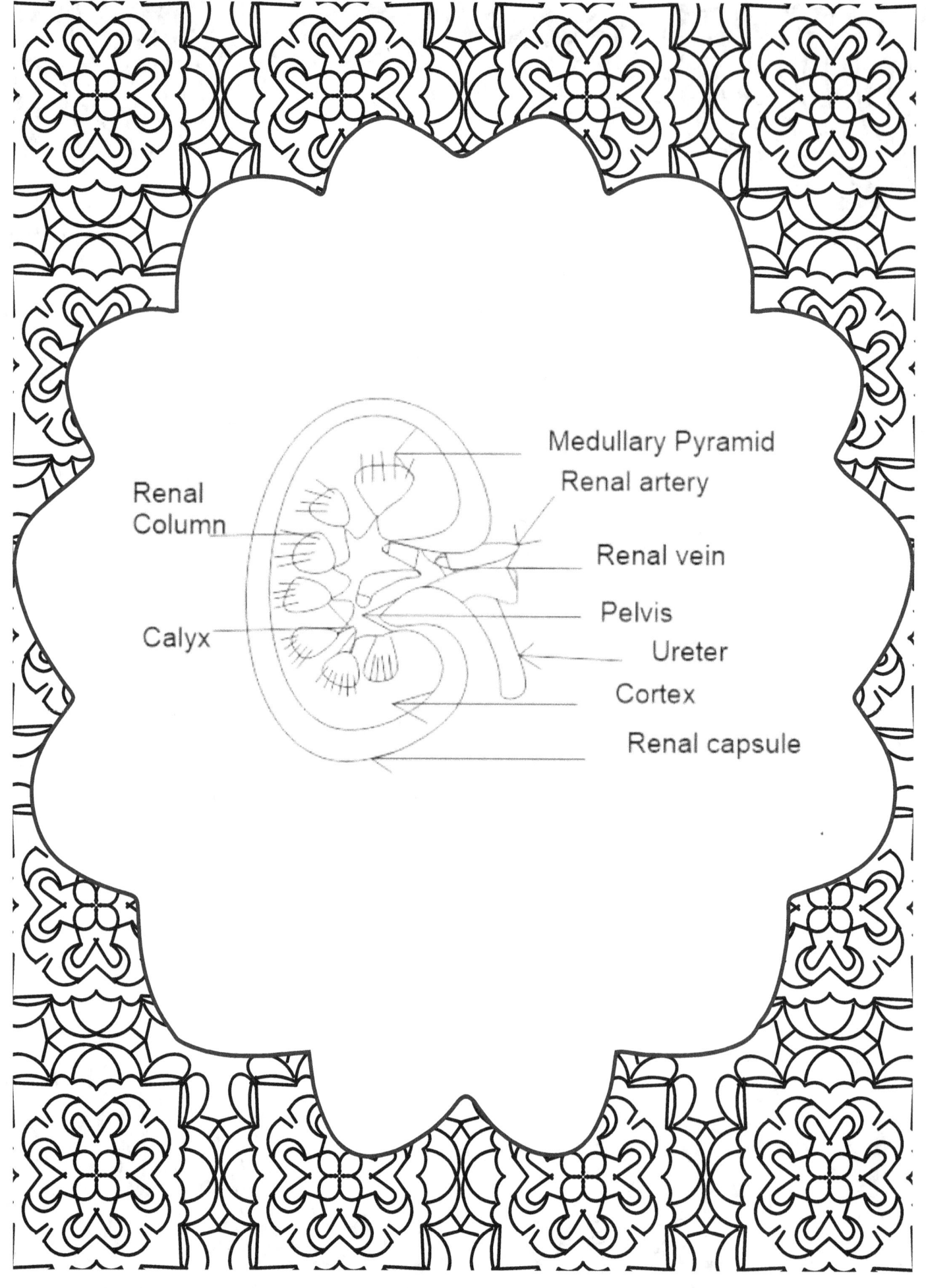

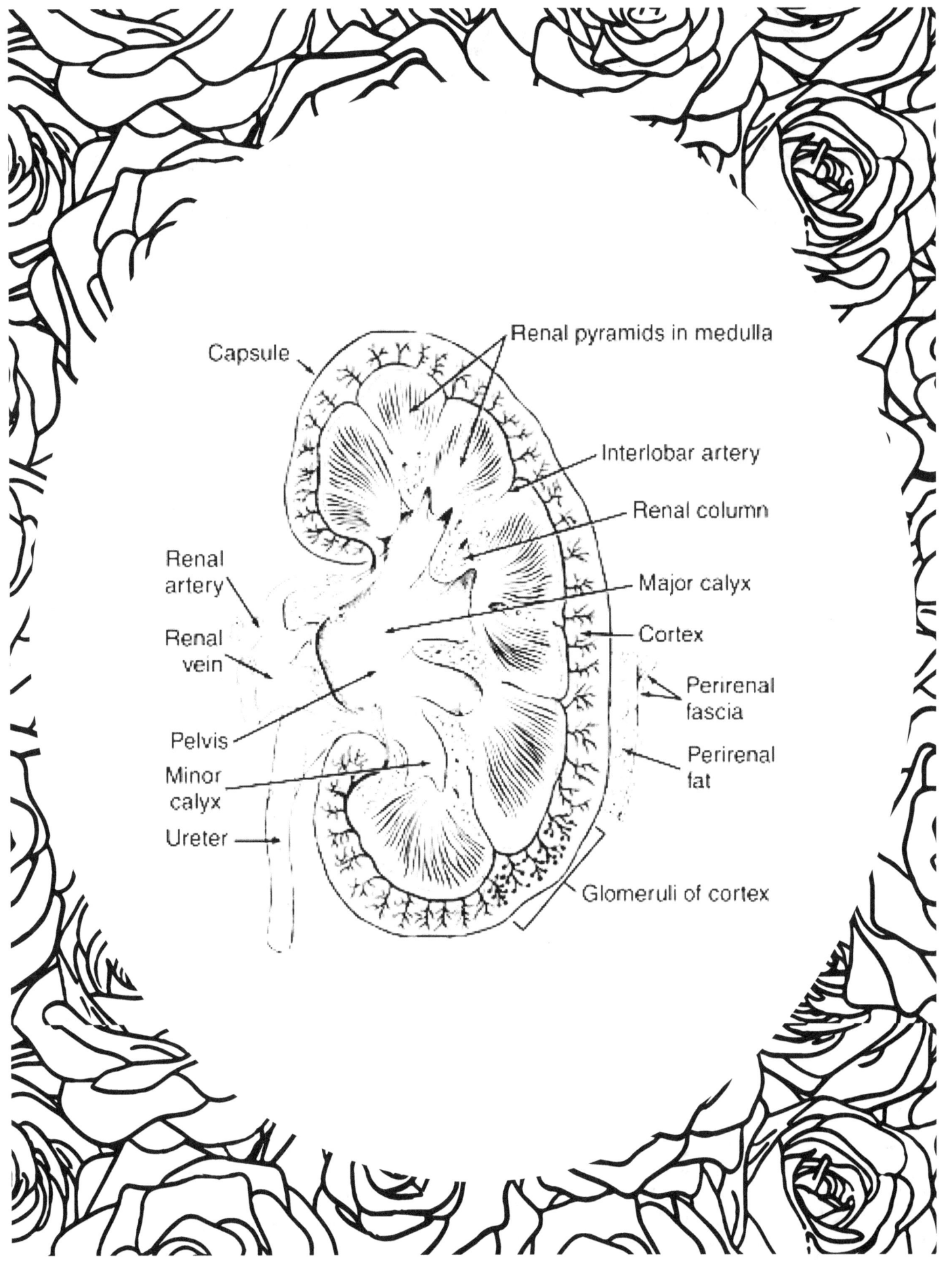

Capsule

Renal pyramids in medulla

Interlobar artery

Renal column

Renal artery

Major calyx

Renal vein

Cortex

Perirenal fascia

Pelvis

Perirenal fat

Minor calyx

Ureter

Glomeruli of cortex

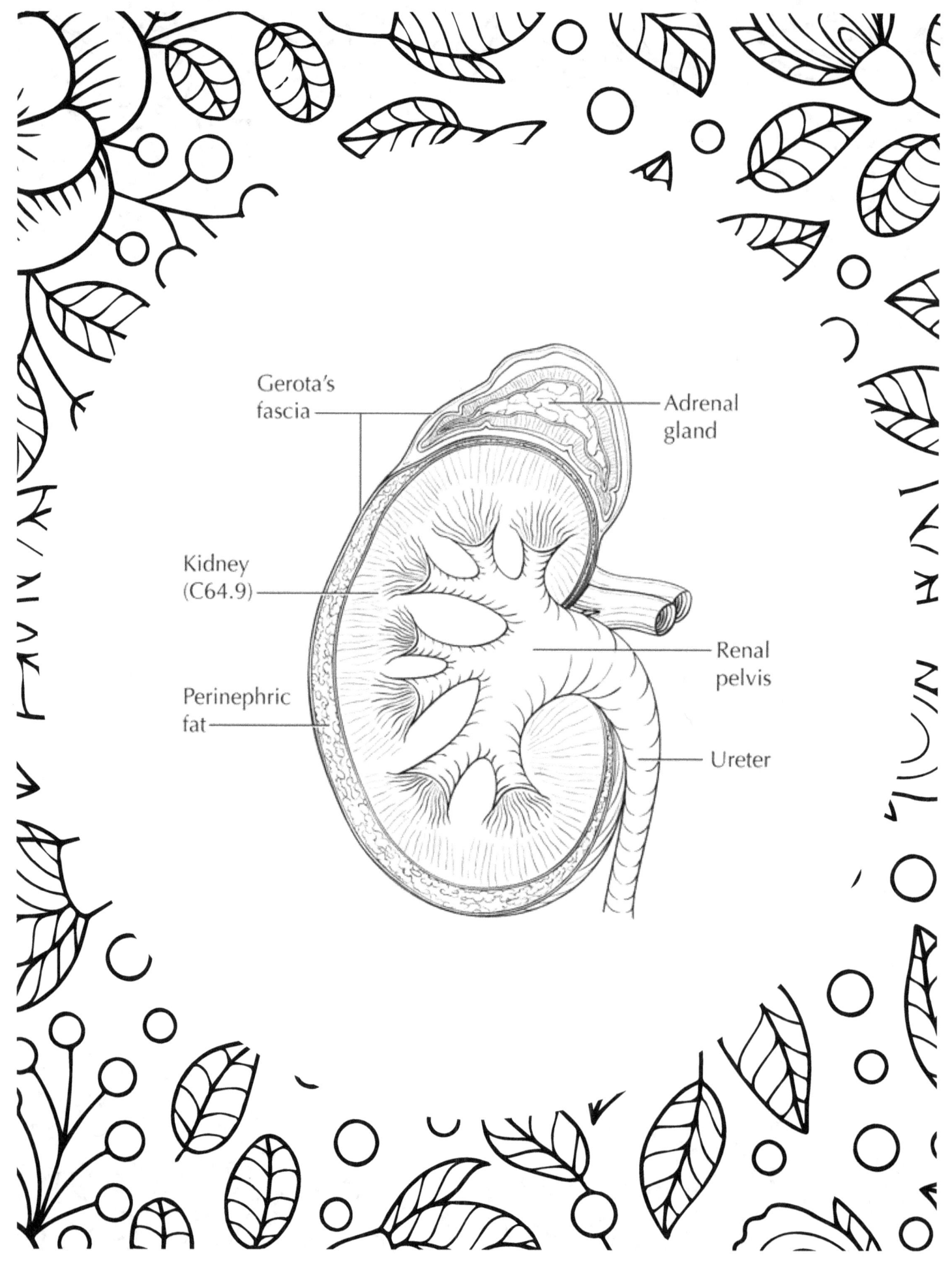

Gerota's fascia

Adrenal gland

Kidney (C64.9)

Renal pelvis

Perinephric fat

Ureter

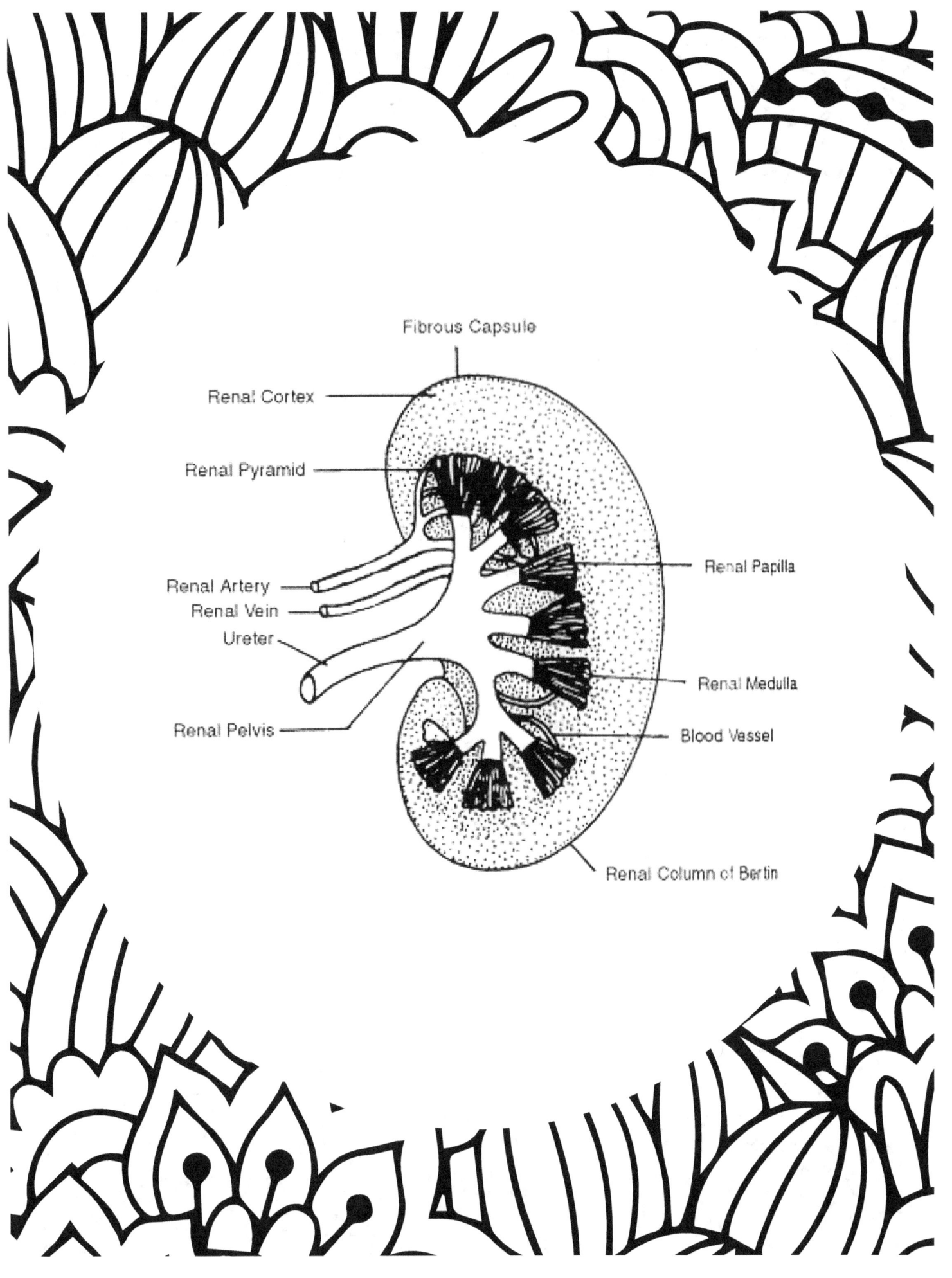

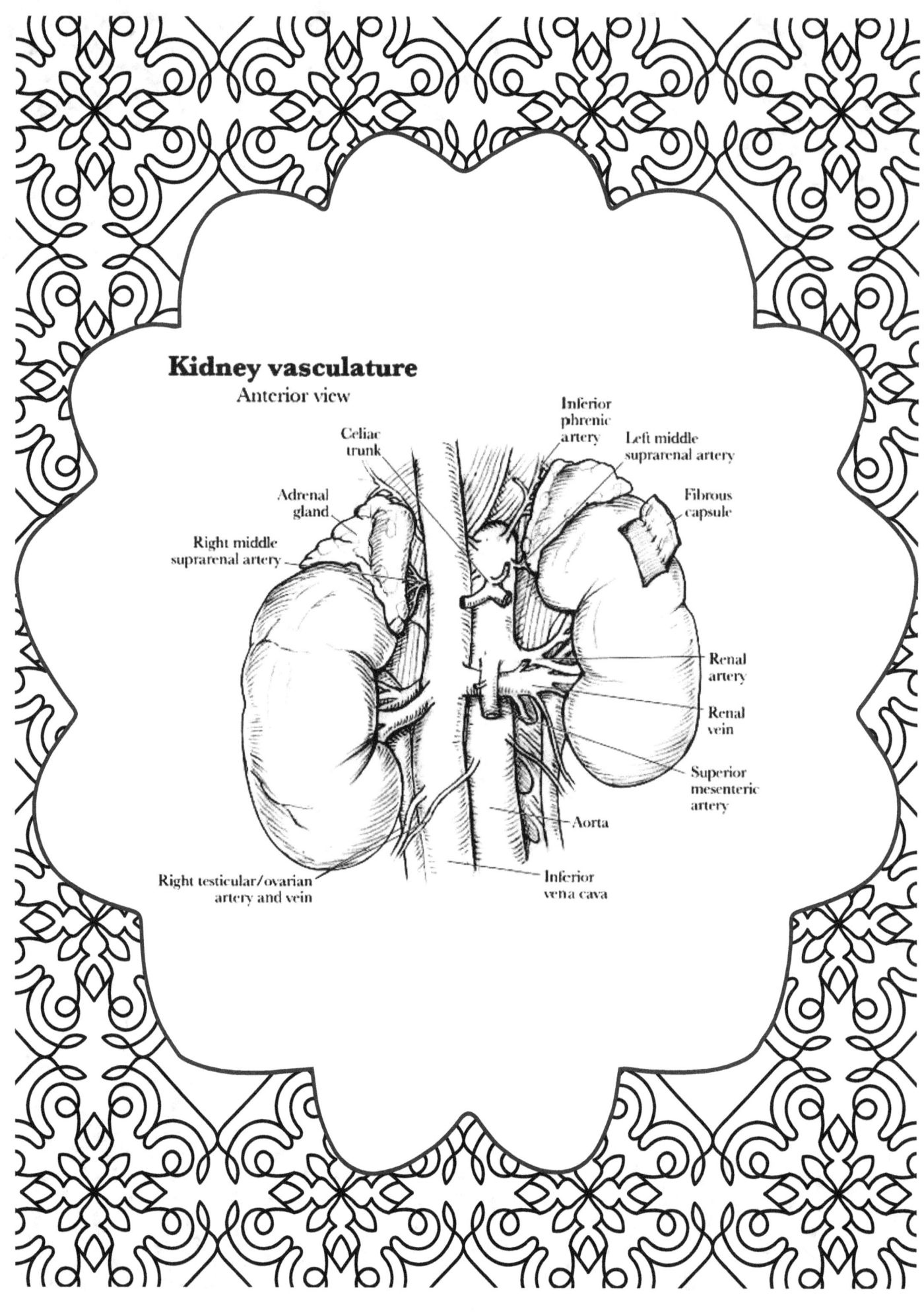

Kidney vasculature
Anterior view

Celiac trunk

Adrenal gland

Right middle suprarenal artery

Inferior phrenic artery

Left middle suprarenal artery

Fibrous capsule

Renal artery

Renal vein

Superior mesenteric artery

Aorta

Inferior vena cava

Right testicular/ovarian artery and vein

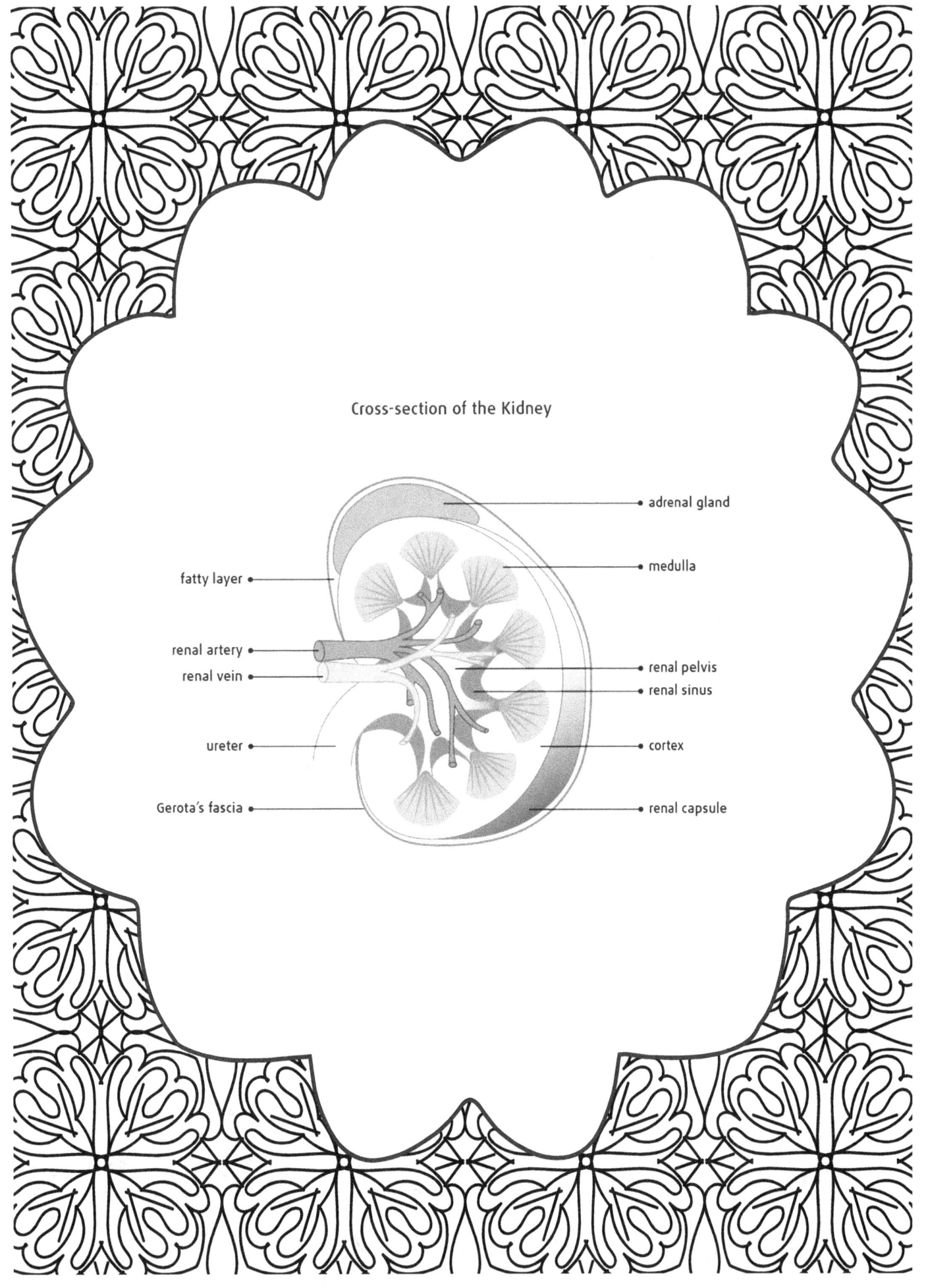

Cross-section of the Kidney

adrenal gland

medulla

fatty layer

renal artery

renal vein

renal pelvis

renal sinus

ureter

cortex

Gerota's fascia

renal capsule

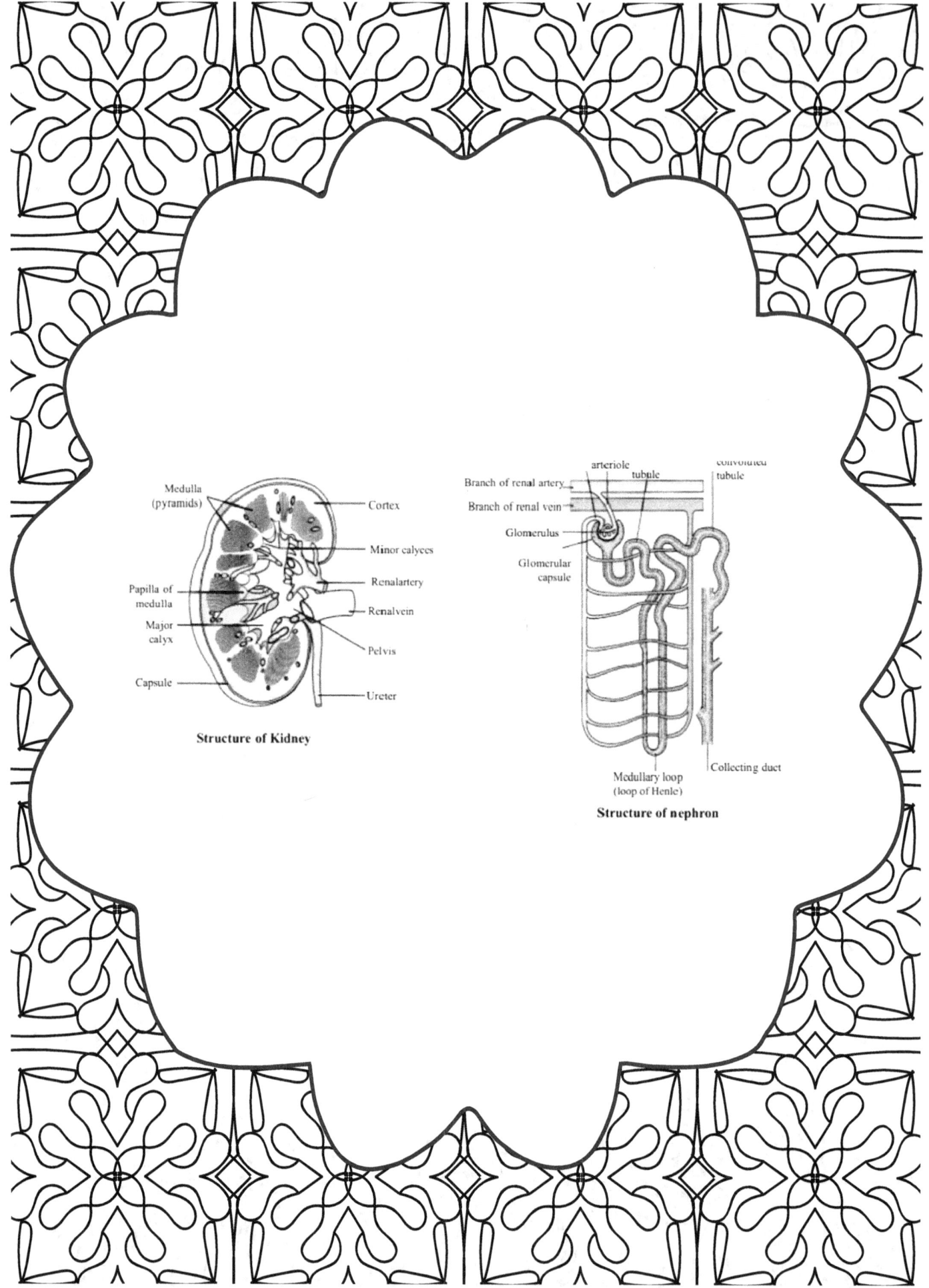

Structure of Kidney

Medulla (pyramids)
Cortex
Minor calyces
Papilla of medulla
Renalartery
Major calyx
Renalvein
Pelvis
Capsule
Ureter

Structure of nephron

arteriole
tubule
convoluted tubule
Branch of renal artery
Branch of renal vein
Glomerulus
Glomerular capsule
Medullary loop (loop of Henle)
Collecting duct

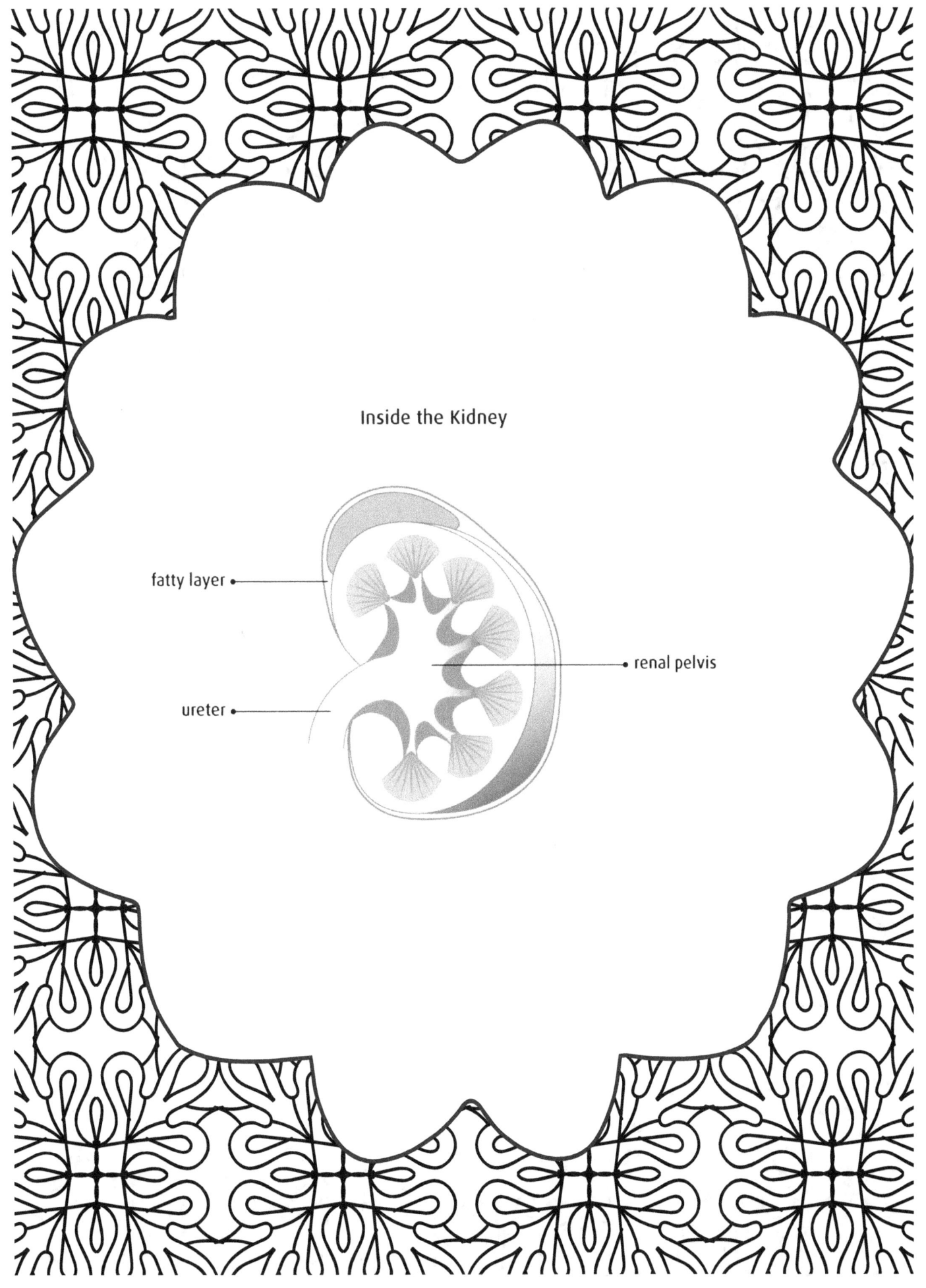

Inside the Kidney

fatty layer

renal pelvis

ureter

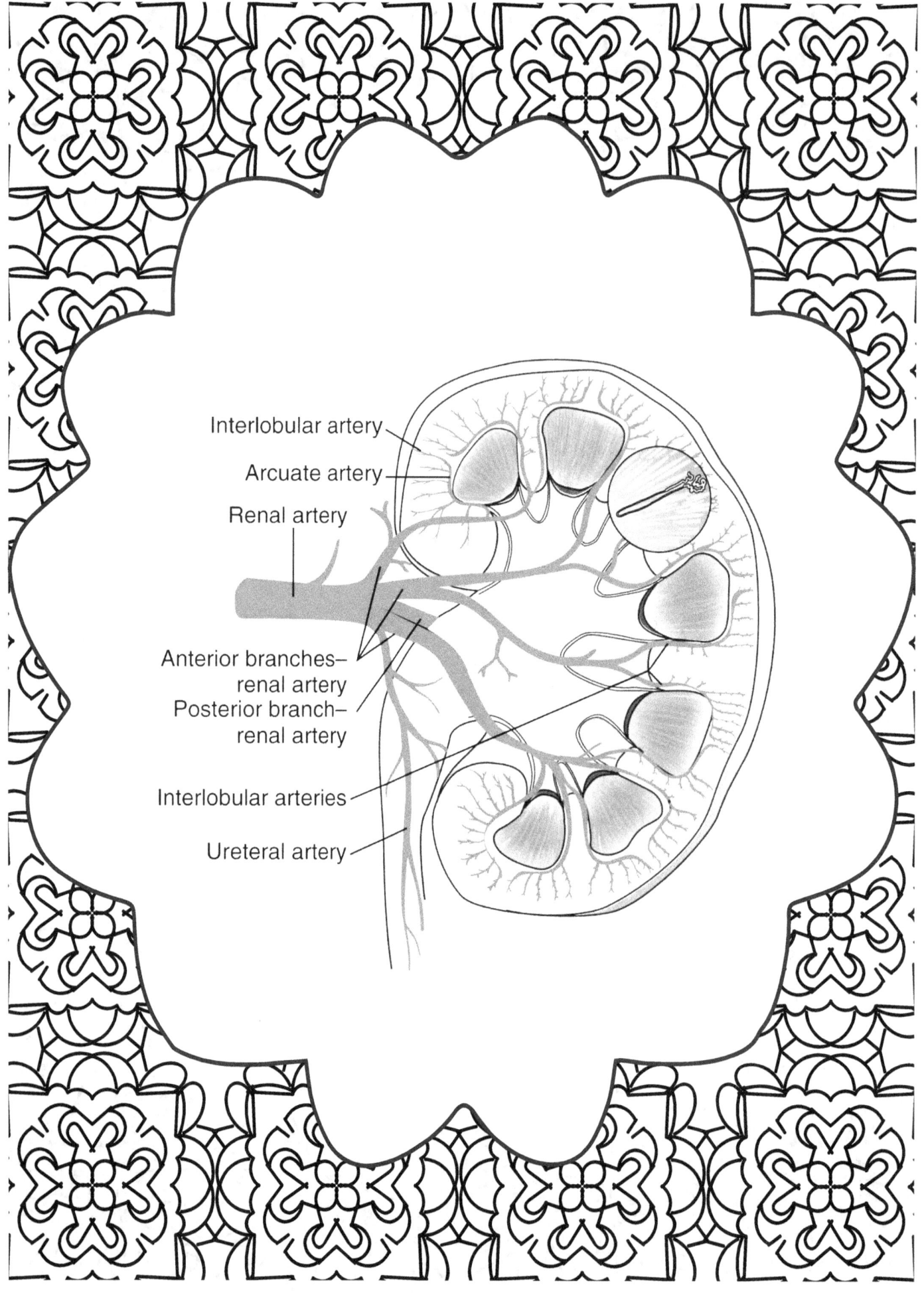

Interlobular artery

Arcuate artery

Renal artery

Anterior branches–
renal artery

Posterior branch–
renal artery

Interlobular arteries

Ureteral artery

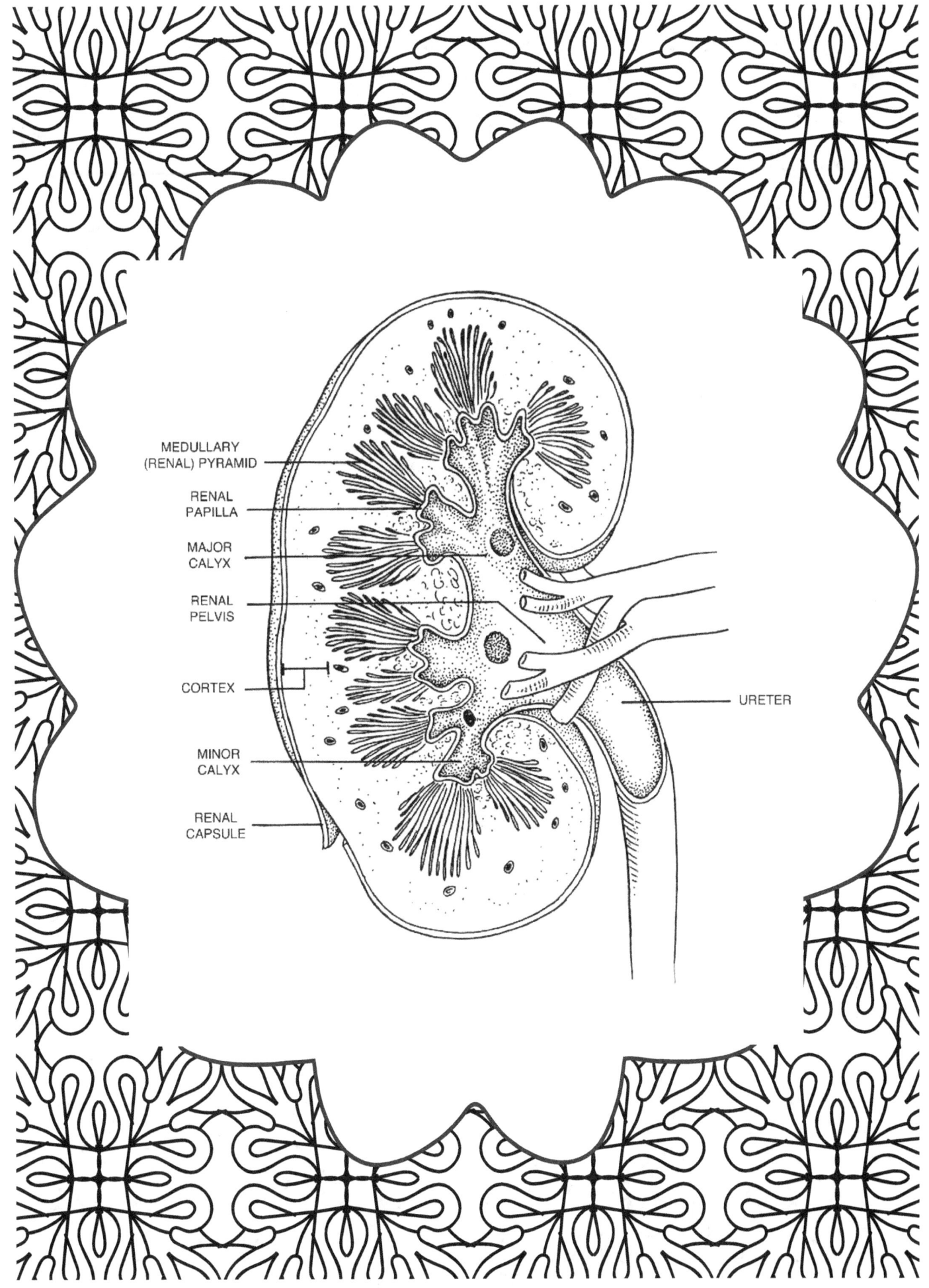

MEDULLARY
(RENAL) PYRAMID

RENAL
PAPILLA

MAJOR
CALYX

RENAL
PELVIS

CORTEX

MINOR
CALYX

RENAL
CAPSULE

URETER

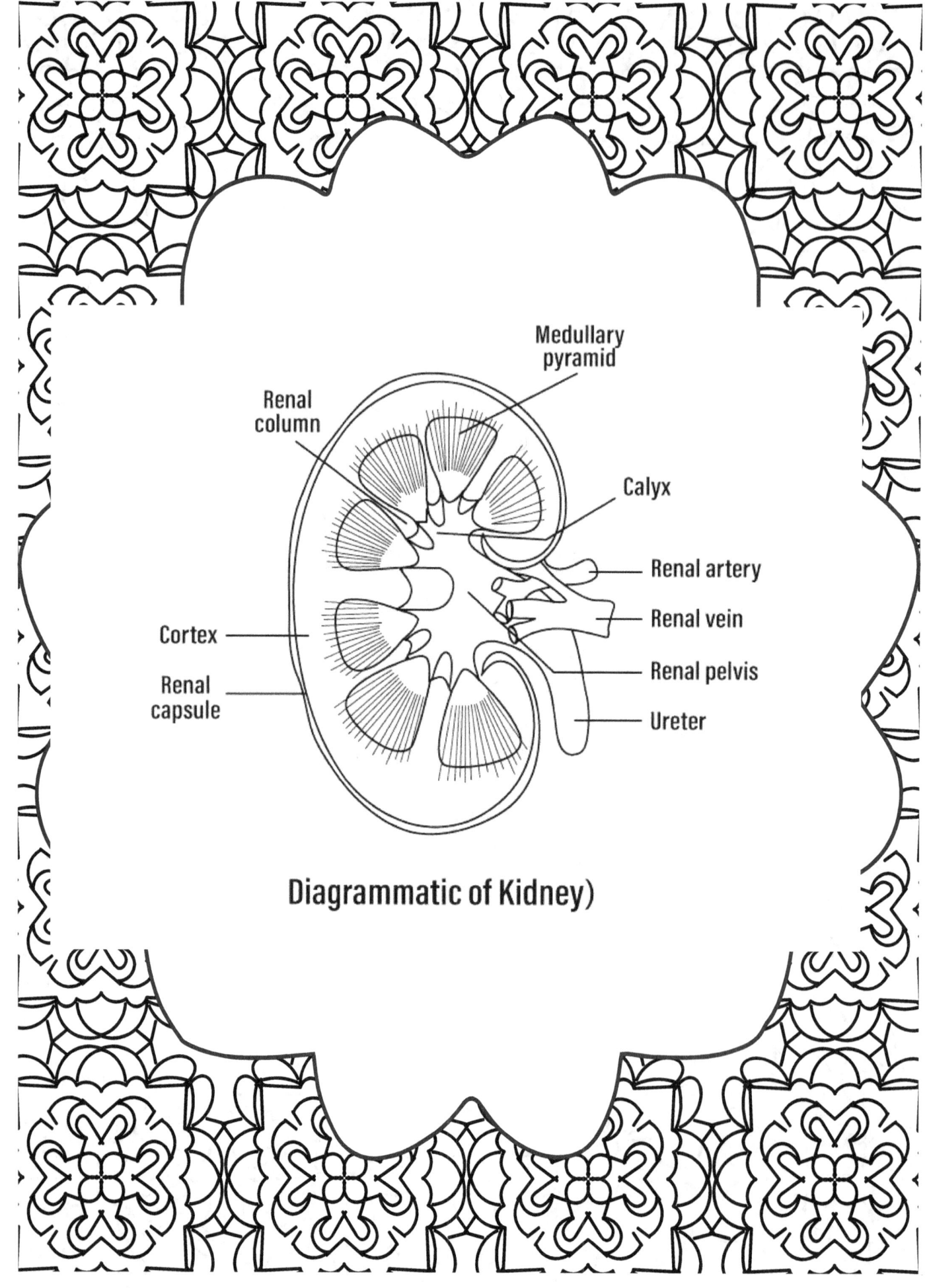

Diagrammatic of Kidney)

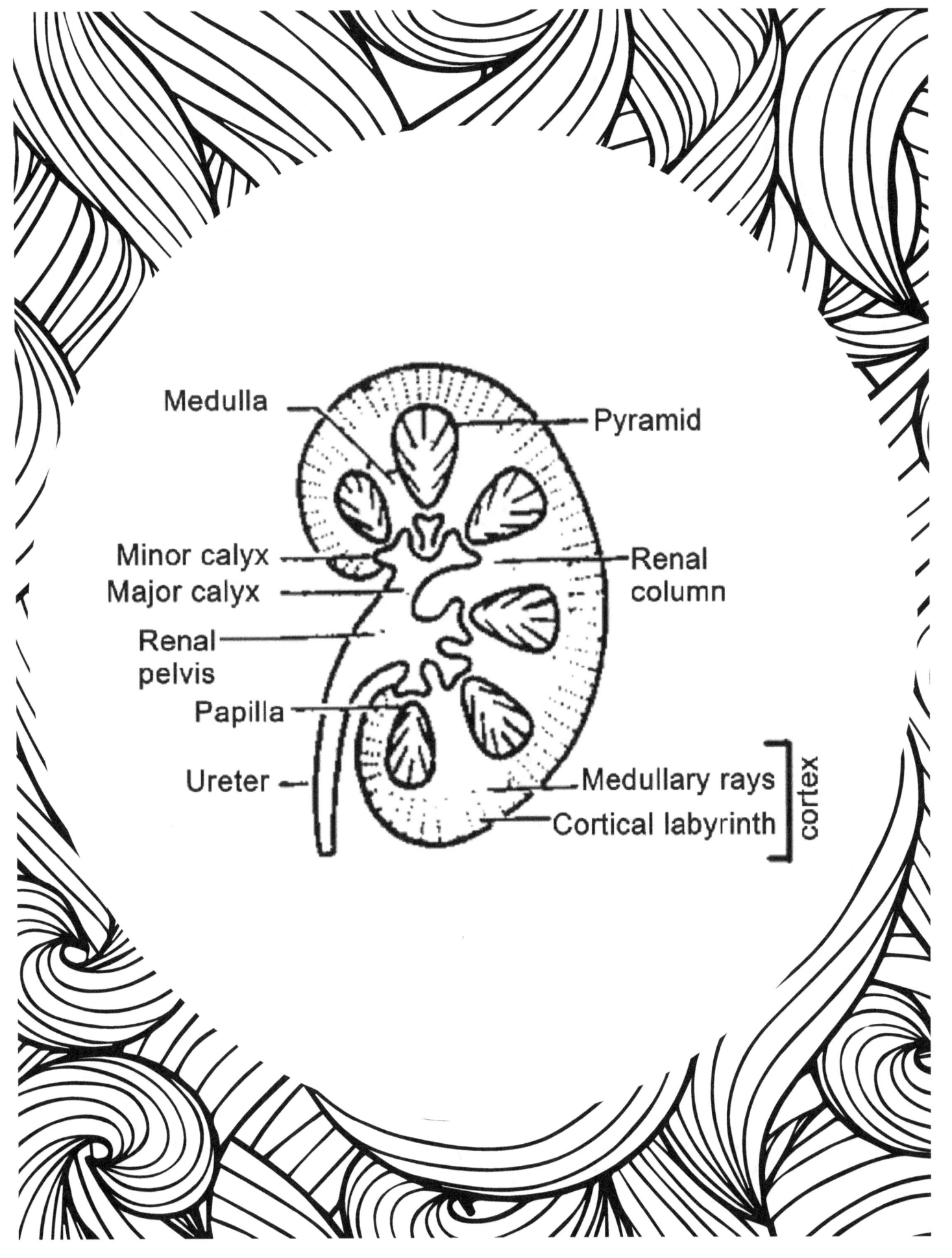

Medulla

Pyramid

Minor calyx

Major calyx

Renal pelvis

Papilla

Ureter

Renal column

Medullary rays

Cortical labyrinth

cortex

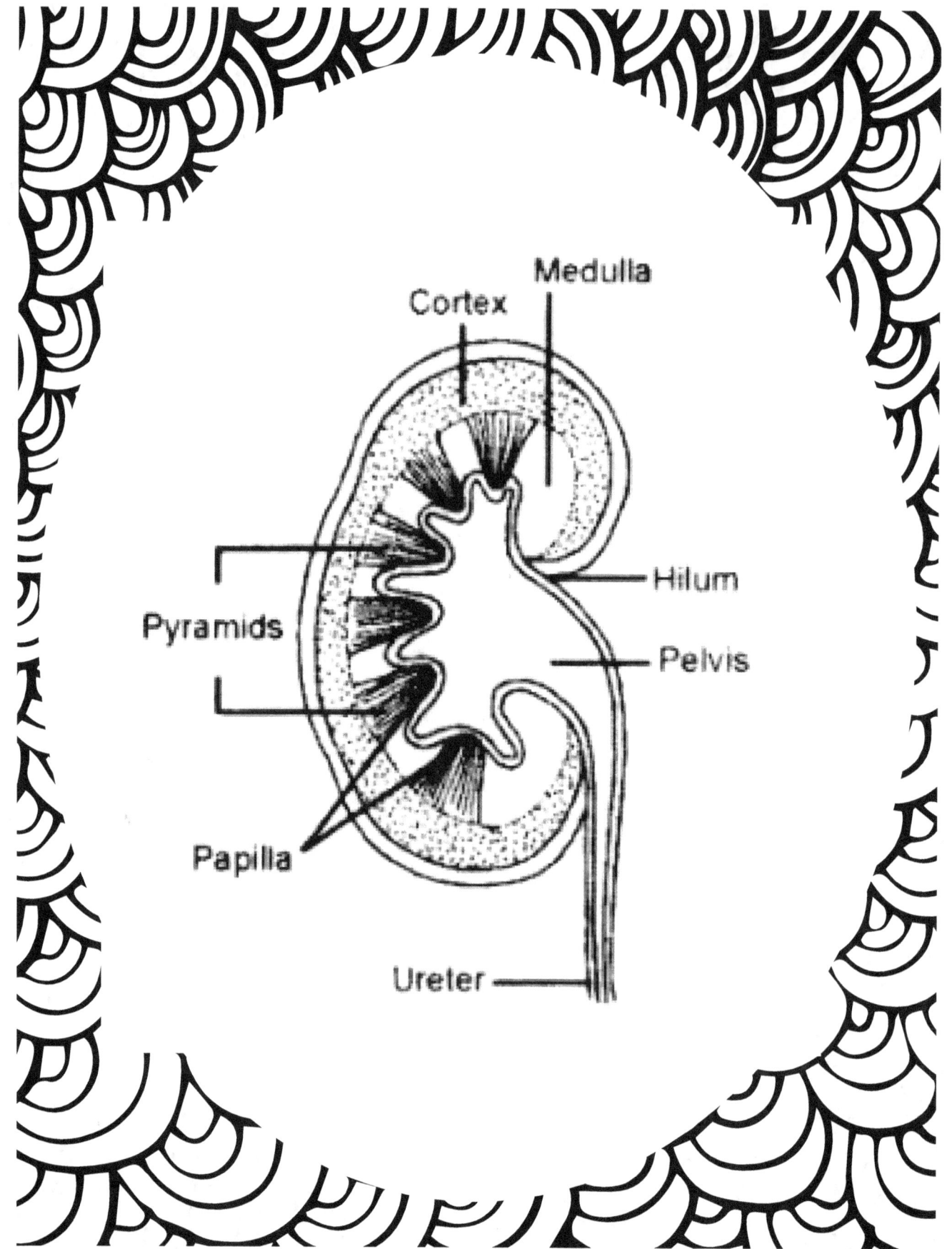

Kidneys and Urinary Tract

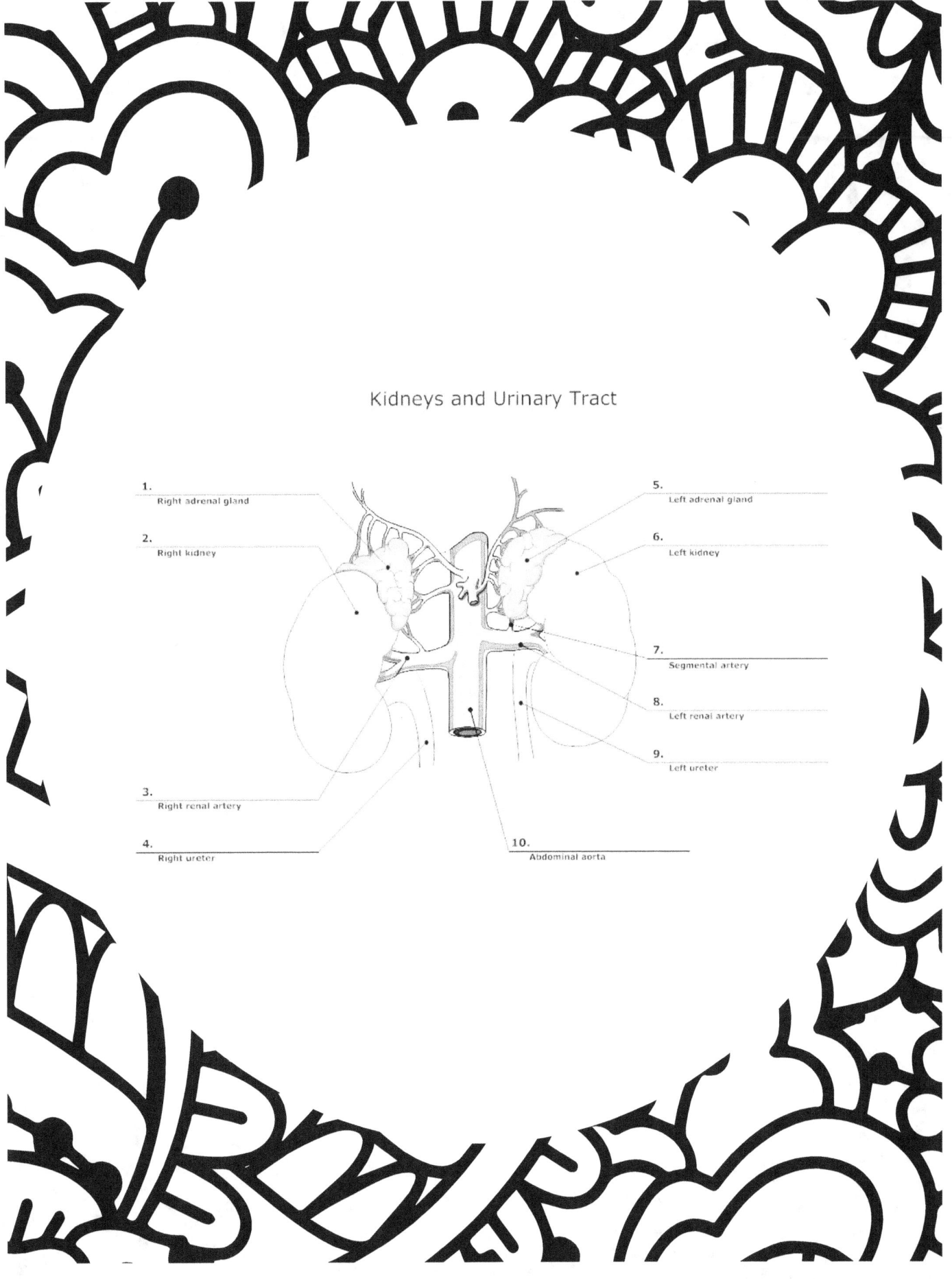

1. _____
   Right adrenal gland

2. _____
   Right kidney

3. _____
   Right renal artery

4. _____
   Right ureter

5. _____
   Left adrenal gland

6. _____
   Left kidney

7. _____
   Segmental artery

8. _____
   Left renal artery

9. _____
   Left ureter

10. _____
    Abdominal aorta

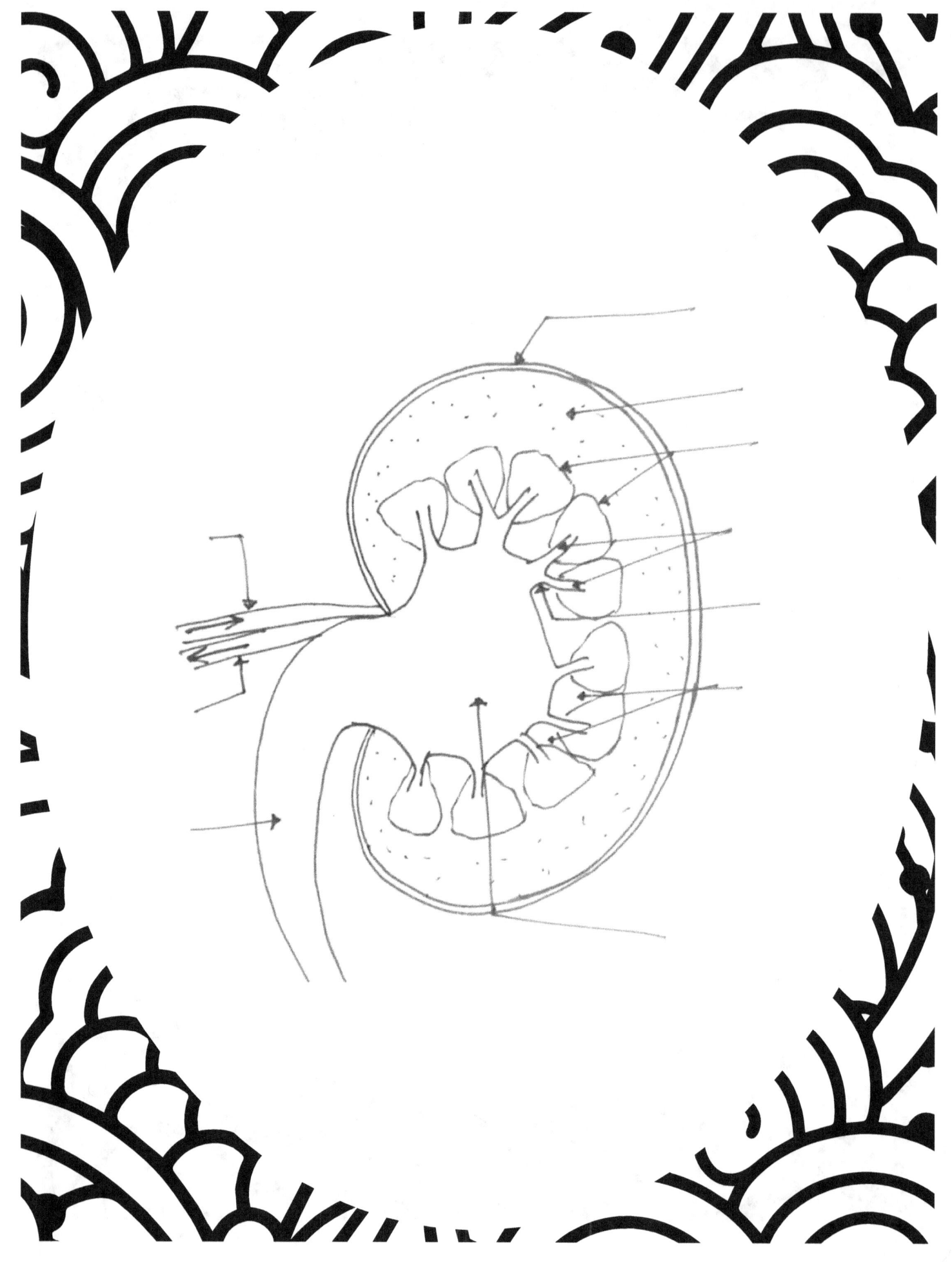

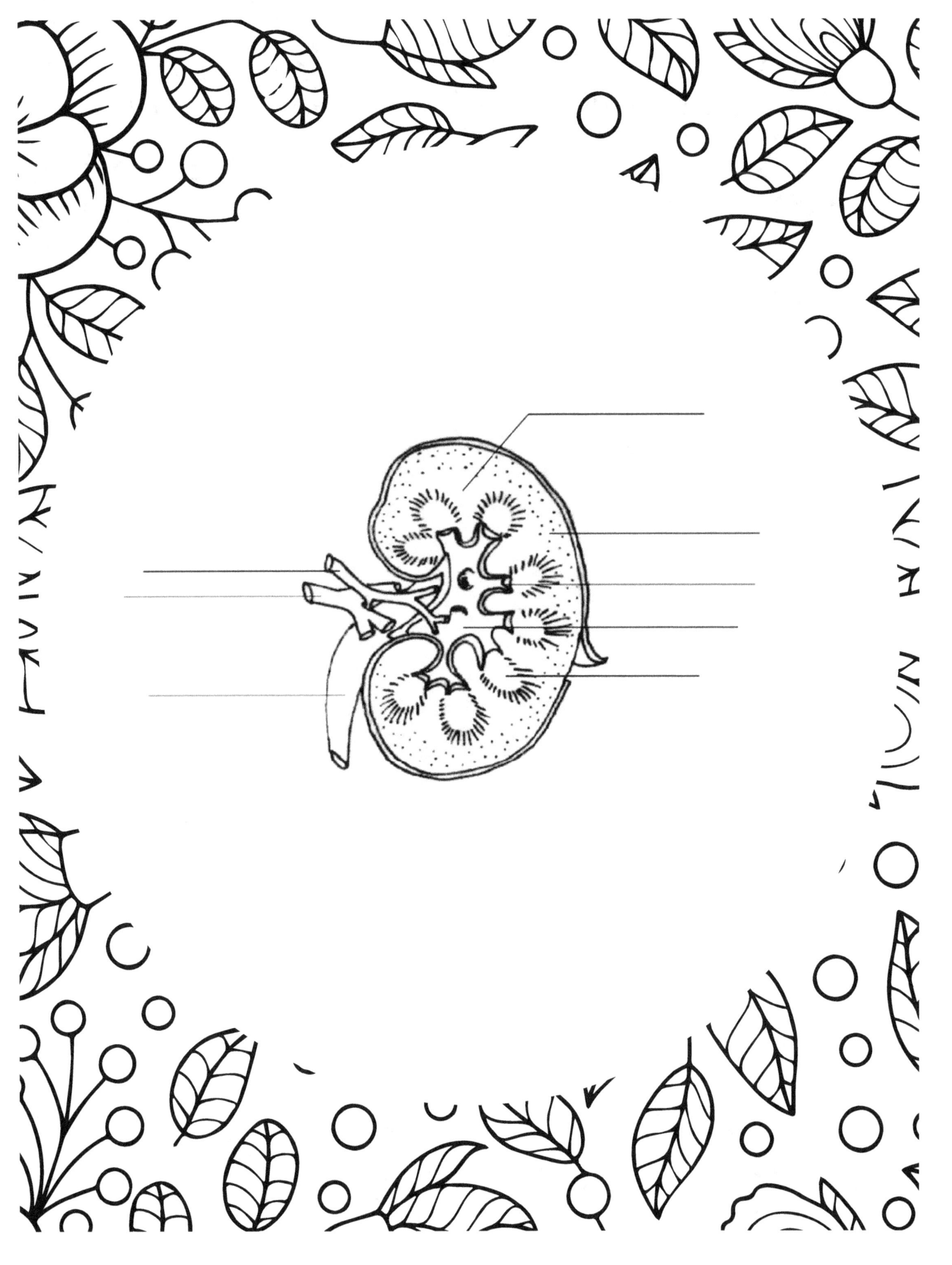

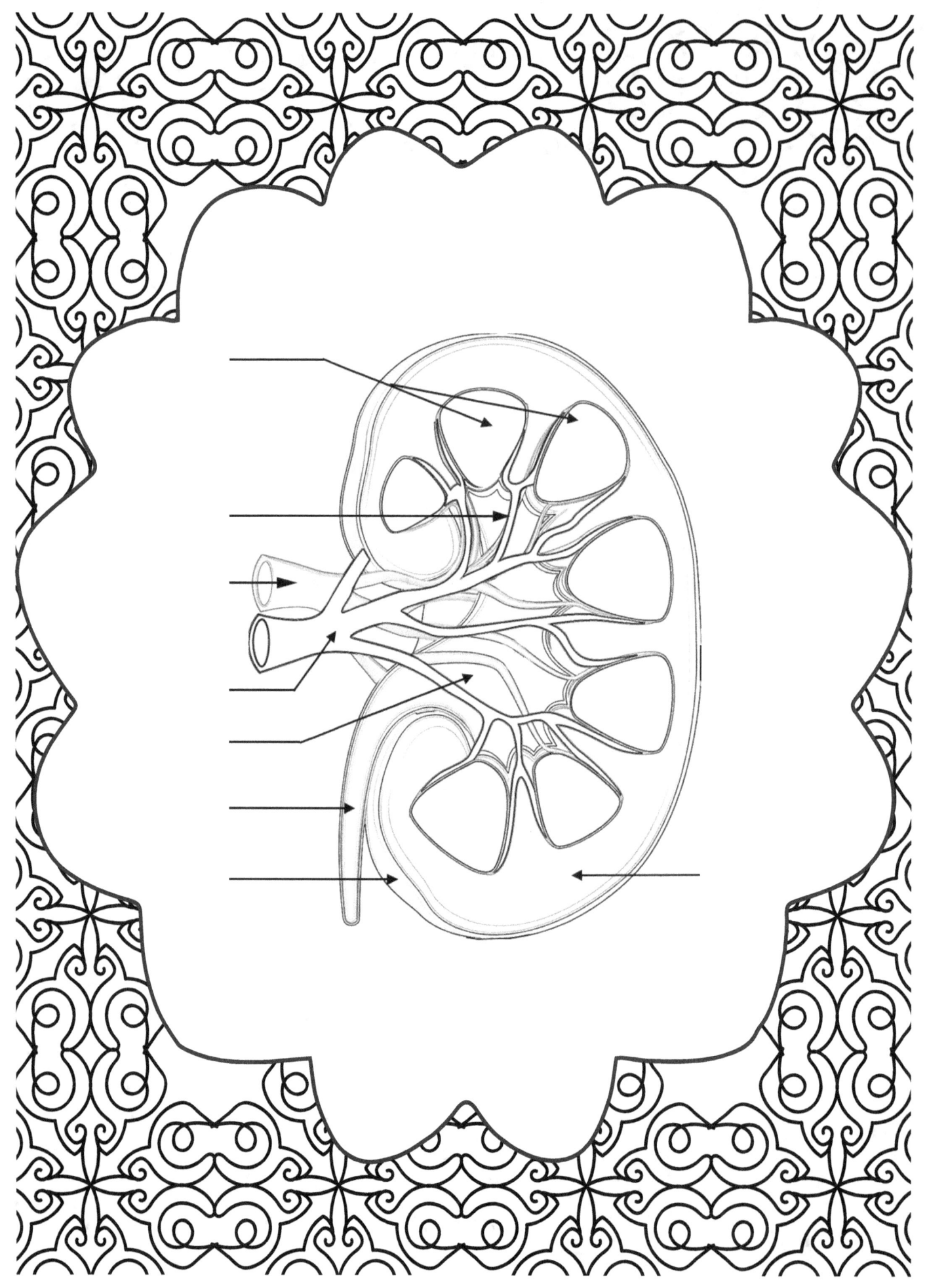